PRAISE FOR

C000183885

Moving and deeply emotional

HELLO! MAGAZINE

Raw, truthful and brave

CAROL DRINKWATER, AUTHOR, *THE OLIVE FARM*

Bold, brave and brilliantly readable

CAROLINE NORRIS, PRODUCER, *MOTHERLAND*

Recommended summer reading

ROSIE NIXON, AUTHOR: *THE STYLIST, JUST BETWEEN FRIENDS*

Exhilarating – I was hooked

NEAL FOSTER, DIRECTOR, BIRMINGHAM STAGE COMPANY

Its power lies in the honesty of her writing

BOOKS ARE MY CWTCHES

Inspiring and relatable

Copyright © Lisa Edwards 2022

This is a work of creative nonfiction. The events are portrayed to the best of the author's memory. While all the stories in this book are true, some names and identifying details have been changed to protect the privacy of the people involved.

Cover design: Clare Baggaley

Publisher: Redwood Tree Publishing Ltd

ISBN (ebook): 978-1-7399340-7-1

ISBN (paperback): 978-1-7399340-8-8

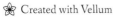 Created with Vellum

DARK HORSES RIDE

ONE WOMAN'S JOURNEY INTO MIDLIFE AND MENOPAUSE

LISA EDWARDS

For Sudhir Rishi, who has changed my life and countless others' through his teachings.

FOREWORD

In 2019 my life was transformed in India and that story is told in my first book, *Cheat Play Live*. I was fifty-two. Before that trip, my second to South Goa, I had lived almost a whole lifetime grieving for my parents and trying to numb that pain with increasing amounts of alcohol. I had married the wrong man because I was trying to do what I thought I should be doing at thirty-five, rather than what was best for me, and for him. At the same time, I was trying to climb a career ladder in publishing that was determined to throw me off it, and struggling inside a viper's nest of toxicity.

My time in Goa showed me that a happy life without a drink in my hand, a man at my side or a high-flying career was possible. It showed me that the love and joy I'd craved since I was a little girl was already inside me and I didn't need to get it from anyone else (although I could, and I did). It introduced 'Little Lisa', my inner child, to the world and let her run free on the sand. It showed me that a life could be lived directed by myself and no one else. I could be in the world, happy and free, just like the White Horse I met every day on the beach.

Once I'd reinvented myself as a freelance editor, writer and qualified yoga teacher, I went back to Goa to see how I might live as a digital nomad. Some might say, and many did, that I was 'living the dream', but what I didn't expect, after White Horse had shown me what freedom looked like, was that Dark Horses would be riding into view right behind her...

All the sun long it was running,
it was lovely, the hay
Fields high as the house, the tunes
from the chimneys, it was air
And playing, lovely and watery
And fire green as grass.
And nightly under the simple stars
As I rode to sleep the owls were bearing
the farm away,
All the moon long I heard, blessed among stables,
the nightjars
Flying with the ricks, and the horses
Flashing into the dark.

Fern Hill, Dylan Thomas

LIVING THE DREAM
INDIA

AGONDA, SOUTH GOA
NOVEMBER 2019

I RUN ACROSS THE POTHOLED ROAD, PULLING MY SUITCASE behind me onto the central reservation, and am narrowly missed by an oncoming lorry and a beeping scooter.

Mr Happy is gesturing to me from across the road. "Come, come!"

"I am coming!" Just as soon as this stream of traffic gets out of the way...

I smile to myself. Only in an Indian airport would you be expected to run across a busy road with your luggage to get to your taxi.

"Oh my god..." Mr Happy isn't happy.

I can see the red battery light flashing on the dashboard but decide not to say anything. Instead, I grin to myself again, knowing this is all part of the experience. I watch Mr Happy turn the ignition key over and over.

"Let's go!" he finally shouts, as the engine shudders into action and he backs slowly into the face of oncoming traffic.

My smile morphs into a set of gritted teeth as cars, lorries and scooters screech all round us, beeping their horns.

I've done this journey from the airport to Agonda before in the darkness of the early hours, but this is the first time I've done it in the late afternoon, when people are still awake. As we drive on, I recognise the painted bus shelters with their advertisements for petrol and Coca Cola and the Catholic churches and Hindu shrines that form the landmarks in each town. This time the shops aren't shuttered – they are throwing light onto the pavements, showing groups of men discussing the day's events over chai or schoolgirls with their hair in plaits, giggling.

As usual, the sides of the road are dotted with dogs, strutting along looking like they have somewhere to go to; or lying directly in the road itself, surprised to find themselves regularly disturbed by a vehicle.

Mr Happy avoids them all deftly. "Is everything ok?" he asks, taking his eyes off the road for moment.

"Yes, I'm ok. I'm impressed with your driving!"

Mr Happy grins, batting his long, dark eyelashes and looking askance at the newly purchased rainbow-coloured dreamcatcher dangling from his rear-view mirror. I suddenly remember that my yoga friend, Chris, calls them 'flycatchers'.

Mr Happy is a taxi driver and local businessman from Agonda. His family own a hut resort in the town. He is called Mr Happy because his name is Anandu, which means 'bliss' in Sanskrit. He is the right person to bring me back to the place I love so much: my other 'home' in South Goa.

Finally, the car lurches out of second gear into third and I exhale with relief. Driving in a low gear in this world of driving obstacles, it feels like I've had to hold my breath for too long.

"I can't believe people overtake on a bend here!" I cry, holding onto the sides of my seat.

"Yes, it is very, very bad," says Mr Happy, calmly.

He pushes the car back down into first gear on the hill and proceeds to overtake a brightly coloured lorry on a bend. The driver in the cab waves him forward, obviously able to see the road ahead. A sign on his bumper says, 'BLOW HORN OK'. Mr Happy beeps in gratitude. I breathe again.

As we turn into the road to Agonda, I spot the empty tables on the corner where women sell fruit and vegetables during the day. I am nearly home and I sigh happily.

"You recognise this place?" Mr Happy asks.

"Yes, I know exactly where we are. We are nearly in Agonda!"

Before dropping me off at my lodgings, Mr Happy pulls up outside his house where his children surround the car, smiling shyly through the windows at me. I get out of the car and they take turns to shake my hand.

Mr Happy turns to his wife, who is approaching in a fuschia-pink patterned sari. "She said she was impressed with my driving," he cries, pointing at me. "I did not tell her that my brakes were not working!"

———

My home for the next six months would be the Red House. It sat grandly in the middle of the main road in Agonda, a Portuguese-style villa with crimson walls and white paintwork. I'd known during my last visit to the village that I would stay here – it called to me every time I walked past. It was near the bar I frequented, Kopi Desa, and there was a convenient sandy path down to the beach right next to it. It was technically the Red Shade Guest House, but I liked its shortened name: the Red House. Simple and to the point.

I'd last been in the village six months earlier. Agonda had worked its way into my soul like no place before it and I knew that I had found a home and family here. I'd also found a strong connection with a young man, Shubham, who worked at Kopi Desa. I was back to see if our virtual romance – one we'd kept going over video message while he was on a cruise ship and I was back in London – was something that could exist in the real world.

I was also here to embark on a new working life – I'd be one of those 'digital nomads' I'd always envied, which would see me freelancing from my laptop in India, wifi-allowing. I'd had my misgivings – at fifty-two, I was supposed to be thinking about settling down into a nice comfy armchair somewhere in the UK and starting to enjoy the fruits of my labours in the publishing industry, but that hadn't been my destiny. For one thing, I couldn't afford to stop working. Fruits were in short supply.

In May 2019, I'd completed my yoga-teacher training and my first book in Agonda. I returned back to my flat in London that summer with a mission in mind: I would not try and seek out another senior role in publishing where I'd spent the last twenty-five years of my career – I would embrace freelance life. For one thing, I knew that such roles would be scarce. I'd seen far too many women like me get pushed off the career ladder in their fifties and I had a sense of what would happen: I would go into circulation as a maternity-cover filler-person and pop up at publishing houses all over London. The children's books scene was peppered with us – women who had been 'someone' in the industry back in the day but had been pushed off the ladder (usually by another woman) in our fifties.

As a publishing director, I'd had these women on my

teams from time to time, and as I got older, I began to realise that there was a very real chance I would become one of them. I wouldn't play the corporate game in a toxic workplace – and ultimately, that would be my downfall; I refused to support ideas and practices that I didn't agree with. So, when my time did come, on a crisp, clear end-of-February day, I turned my face to the sun as I walked back home through Holland Park and knew exactly what to do: I would return to India and embark on a spiritual journey.

Three months later, I set about packing up my home, putting everything in storage and renting out my flat to enable me to go back and live in India for six months. Because I could. I had no ties (an ex-husband, no kids and a dwindling number of family) and I wanted to start a new life away from city life, from the lure of the London publishing scene and its drinking culture. I was in my first year of sobriety, having had my last drink in Goa in January 2019.

Once I made that decision, I felt an incredible urge to get rid of stuff; shedloads of it. I'd had to do it once before when I'd left my marital home nine years earlier, and moved out of a four-bedroomed house in Buckinghamshire into a one-bedroomed flat in the city. Then, as now, it gave me great pleasure to slough off everything that had formed my previous life.

The first time it had been an exodus of shared marital possessions – a peeling sofa that had to go to a skip; the mountain bike I'd never really wanted that got stolen. It was as though these things knew they were no longer wanted, so they fell into ruin or disappeared from my life without any effort from me. Gradually, I'd replaced them with things that were mine and mine only. But now I could see that I was still holding on to possessions that I didn't need. I could only afford a small storage pod so I had to make decisions on what had to go. Quickly, a 'get-rid' plan emerged.

I started by extracting a selection of books from my huge collection and made piles of them in the lobby of the 'gold building' where I lived among fifty other flats in Kensal Rise, north-west London. I posted on our Facebook group that they were free to whomever wanted them and half an hour later, they'd all gone. I still had bulging shelves of books but I couldn't quite part with my collections of Murakami, Theroux and all the other authors I loved. I don't know why getting rid of books is the hardest thing to do, but all I know is, I'm still paying for a small library to sit in storage. They form the bulk of my possessions, along with fake-leather photo albums filled with all the holiday photos from my failed marriage.

I went through all my toiletries and beauty products and put everything I'd been hanging onto – tiny sample bottles of serum I kept for no reason, the shampoo for hair I no longer coloured, the palettes of eyeshadow I kept for a 'you never know' moment even though I'd largely stopped wearing make-up – into a tub and placed it in the lobby. Again, every-thing went, taken by the gold building's unseen elves.

My desire to declutter gained momentum – I experi-enced an actual rush whenever I was cleansed of another set of things I didn't need: clothes in the wrong size that I was keeping for the day I would be the right size; numerous bottles of alcohol; an ugly glass TV table and a huge collec-tion of CDs that couldn't be played on anything – the more I got rid of, the more I could see another layer of unnecessary belongings around me.

I started to post items for pick-up on Facebook Market-place and met wonderful people who really would give my things a good home. A man picked up my camera for his daughter for her school projects; a woman took my entire DVD collection to cheer her auntie up after losing her husband (I didn't have the heart to tell her that most of them were stories of heartbreak with tragic endings). A Brazilian family picked up my beloved iMac – the model with the periscopic head that I'd bought with my first work bonus at the turn of the century. (It turned out that it was the only bonus I actually got in publishing so I'm glad I spent it wisely).

As everything disappeared from my little flat one by one, a lighter, brighter future emerged. I remembered why I'd felt so light and free moving into this flat in the first place, now that the sunlight could bounce off its huge white walls. Why had I felt the need to fill the space again, when the spaces I'd found when I first moved in were so deliciously free of stuff and so liberating?

I enjoyed the countdown of months, then weeks, until my departure for India in November, just as the winter in the UK was about to start. Each week brought a freshly cleared space in my flat and the weights of my past – the unhappy marriage and relationships, the stressful jobs, the alcohol addiction – were lifting. I began to pack my bags and set aside some belongings for my return in six months' time, to be stored at a friend's house. It was more stressful deciding what to keep than deciding what to get rid of – and I knew I wouldn't see my stored things for a long time to come. What could I live without?

On the last night in my flat I slept in a sleeping bag on my stripped bed, with all my worldly goods packed into a large rucksack, suitcase and carry-on pack. Everything else had gone into storage, wedged into a tiny metal box by a huge Ukrainian guy who was determined not to have me paying for a second pod. He beamed proudly when he was done, obviously loving the satisfaction of making everything fit in, as though he'd been playing a giant game of reverse Jenga.

I wake up to the sound of the poder's horn – he is carrying warm bread in a basket for the people in the village and will return again in the evening. The soft light of dawn is streaming in through curtains patterned with palm leaves, and I am lying under a bright-green cotton sheet covered with pink and orange flowers.

The bed is a dark cedar with a thin mattress and plenty of space for my bags underneath, although I can see that the shelving at the top of the opposite wall is probably the best place for them – no creatures seeking sanctuary up there.

My 'wardrobe' is a coat stand, so I drape the dresses I've bought on previous trips here from its hooks and in the morning light I admire all the clashing-print glory of my new abode.

I walk into the bathroom and smile at the pink tiles and feature wall of lotus flowers. I will be happy here.

I pull on denim shorts, a vest and some flip-flops, slathering on factor 50 before doing so – I am pale and sensitive-skinned again after my six months back in the UK. The sun isn't up yet and I don't want to miss its rising glory, over the horizon I've grown to love so much.

I walk out of the house and find my landlord, Marshall, sweeping the courtyard outside the house in the cool morning air.

"You sleep well?" he asks with a shy smile, averting his gaze as though he's caught me in my pyjamas.

"Yes, yes ... I've slept well, thank you."

Of course I have: I'm home.

I pass two sleeping pigs as I walk down the alley to the beach. They are nestled snout to tail, snuffling in their slumber, unaware of me standing staring adoringly at them.

A tiny puppy runs out of the Love Bites café, shaking and weeing in the sand before his owner retrieves him. The puppy's name is Ocean, the young man tells me, rescued in the cyclone a few weeks earlier. "It ripped through the village," he says.

I take my flip-flops off and leave them in the sand outside Agonda Diva resort, in the safe keeping of a sleeping dog who doesn't even open an eye as I pass. The staff are sleeping under cotton sheets on the tables and chairs, the fabric pulled over their heads to stop the mosquitoes from biting.

I step down on to the cool sand and look for my pack – the dogs that I've grown to love on my last visit: Sanjo and Zimbo, and of course, Sweetpea. There are dogs sleeping like doughnuts curled in the sand all along the beach. I spot Sanjo standing up and stretching his legs, his Scooby Doo-like frame visible from far away. Then I wait for a small golden head near him – Zimbo – to look up and notice me.

And then it begins: the Great Run Up. One tiny blonde dog, another giant galumphing one alongside him, running crazily towards me across the golden sand. They skid round me in excitement, Sanjo almost knocking me over. He doesn't know his own strength. He reminds me of someone.

Sherry, Zimbo's sister, trails behind barking, unable to keep up on her arthritic little legs. They all tumble into the surf in front of me, as if inviting me to go in with them. I laugh *as their little bodies are submerged for a moment, and then they prance back onto the sand, shaking. Sanjo stands above them, amused at his little companions, keen to try and knock me over again.*

But where is Sweetpea?

The pack follow me to Simrose, where I wrote my first book and found a new 'family' in India. The other dogs stay back as I climb the red steps up to the resort, for under its cedarwood sign, there is my love.

Sweetpea is sitting sentinel at the top, her white-flashed nose, chest and paws lit by the rising morning sun. But something is missing – her signature red collar. I reached out to pat her, but she slinks away under the seats.

Trying not to feel disappointed, I continue to walk the length of the wide beach towards the river in the sea mist, passing men brushing their teeth, staring blankly at the sea, and the fishermen quietly bringing in their catch in woollen hats and thick jackets.

I notice that the beach is unusually strewn with debris, and a high sand 'shelf' has been carved into it by strong waves. Zimbo enjoys the height it has afforded him, running alongside me, finally level with Sanjo.

The dogs suddenly sprint off, chasing a young man riding a mahogany-coloured horse along the shore. The boy looks back at me and laughs as he urges the horse to run faster, leaving the barking dogs in his wake.

On my return I catch up with Dinesh, the manager of Simrose. He is already smartly dressed in his pressed beige shirt and trousers, smiling and ready to greet guests. He hugs me and welcomes me home, telling me my coffee and 'crispy toast' are already in progress. But then he tells me that Sweetpea had been hurt after I left last season.

"I found her under one of our cabanas," he says, clearly still traumatised by it all. "She must have crawled there. She was covered in blood. Her neck had been cut. It was a perfect cut, so we don't think it was another dog. No animal would make a cut like that."

That solved the mystery of the missing red collar: Sweetpea's neck was too sore to wear it. Dinesh had taken her to the incredible Brendy at Animal Rescue Agonda, who had kept her there and cared for her until she was well enough to go back to Simrose. Brendy told me later that the cut was likely to have been made by barbed wire; perhaps Sweetpea had crawled under a fence. She knew the locals and knew they would never deliberately cut a dog's neck.

Sweetpea was back, but the light in her eyes had gone out and she seemed lacklustre and low. Another dog had taken over her territory – a small, fox-like animal – and she barked at him weakly from her position under the restaurant seats. *Poor Sweetpea.*

Dinesh told me that the whole of Agonda, including Simrose, was undergoing a major repair programme following the ravages of Cyclone Kyarr a month earlier. It had reached the intensity of a category 4 hurricane, and was the strongest storm recorded in Goa for twelve years. The winds had reached 155 miles per hour. That explained the huge sand shelf running for most of the length of the beach and the blue tarpaulin sheets draped over some of the restaurants at the back of it.

But there was a storm brewing on land too. The Goa Coastal Zone Management Authority had Agonda under its eye as a turtle-nesting site where no unlicensed property was allowed to be on the beach, and no buildings were allowed to have concrete foundations unless they carried an original Agondan address. Most resorts in the village were constructed for the season and taken down again at the end for the same reason, but some had managed to lay down permanent foundations and they'd had a blind eye turned towards them for years. Until now.

Some establishments managed to get a last-minute stay of execution, but twenty-two shacks were due to be demolished. Two hundred young policemen and women were stationed at various resorts along the strand and diggers were parked threateningly nearby. Despite being the home address of one of Agonda's oldest families, Simrose wasn't yet in the clear. Hurried, worried conversations with men in more pressed beige shirts and slacks were taking place over breakfast in the restaurant. Dinesh hugged me again, happy to see me, but he had to go and make sure everything was ok.

I walked back to the Red House trailing Sanjo and Zimbo behind me, unable to comprehend what I was seeing and hearing. The demolition threat had been hanging over Agonda for years – no one believed it would actually happen ... until it did.

Later that day, I joined the throngs on the beach watching one of the unlicensed resorts get smashed to pieces. It was wanton destruction – newly fitted air-conditioners, modern bathrooms and cedar bedroom furniture lay strewn in the sand. We all stood around on the sand in shock, surrounded by uprooted murders of crows. Tourists started to say they were going to stay in other towns because their favourite bars had gone, using the term '*war zone*' to describe the unfolding scene. My head said that I should probably go with them, but my heart decided that I wasn't going anywhere – Agonda was my home and I would stay with it whatever happened. I wanted to support the businesses that were still standing.

I walked back slowly along the bougainvillea-bordered beach road and was cheered by the sight of a blue cart and my friend Charlie standing behind it, smiling, stirring a pan of chai. "Hello my friend!" he shouted. "Chai?"

I can never say no to chai. A speaker hanging from the cart was playing popular songs in Konkani – the Goan language – its carnival beats and optimistic brass section flinging me headlong from demolition on the beach into a party atmosphere.

I took a seat on one of Charlie's little blue plastic chairs and made small talk. I always struggled with small talk back in the UK but here it was an art form, allowing any subject to pop up unannounced, interrupting the previous one. It didn't matter if you didn't finish the thread – you just moved on. In any case, our conversation was regularly interrupted by people coming to the cart to order their morning samosas with chai. I'd be back for an omelette sandwich on puffy white *pao* bread at lunchtime.

As I left Charlie's cart, I spied my friend Gita standing just inside her shop, her small son behind her, peering round the lime-green jewelled silk kurta hanging stiffly over her red leggings. Her laughter greeted me.

"I have lots of new dresses for you, my friend!" Gita cried, gesturing at the racks of new silk halterneck maxi dresses and matching tops and shorts.

I immediately wanted to buy everything. It was a sea of turquoise and sea greens and blues – my favourites. Gita knew how to reel me in and her dark eyes sparkled at me mischievously. I knew I'd be spending my first Sampoorna Yoga School paycheck there.

I was returning to the school where I'd trained to be a yoga teacher, not only as a regular drop-in student, but also as a writer for their website. Whilst I knew I wasn't the best at yoga, I definitely knew I had a way with words, and looked forward to writing about my new-found passion for yoga, alongside keeping my editorial work going. I had also booked on a Yin Yoga course that would take place for a week at the end of November.

I needed to keep busy because Shubham, the man I'd become seriously attached to over the past year, wasn't back in Goa. He'd boarded a cruise ship back in April and wouldn't be arriving in Agonda for another month. I couldn't wait to see him again – we'd fantasised about the moment in every video call we'd had – but I was happy to have some time for myself, to live and breathe this new life here in a Goan village, and to settle into a new routine of living and working in a whole new way.

Most of my days started with a sunrise beach walk with the pack. If I didn't say hello to Captain Nitesh as he pulled his boat out (often helping him to do so) or see the place where the ocean met the river at the far end of the beach, something didn't feel right.

Most mornings I met Stef, an Italian-Israeli who loved Agonda in the off-season, only coming to the beach in the early hours. He trailed a pack of dogs in his wake, the only one actually owned by him being Luna, a fluffy, white, husky-like dog who must have been permanently boiling hot. She lay down whenever she could and huffed when she was made to move.

Stef talked to all the dogs like they were friends, with

individual personalities and quirks (which is, of course, exactly what they were). He caused havoc on the beach wherever he went because the dogs were unruly and wild, and not really listening to a word he said. He just liked shouting their names as they ran after the boy on the mahogany horse or darted into restaurants and resorts for food.

Stef's take on the 'war zone' in Agonda was that it was a good thing, because it would take the village back to what it used to be: quiet. For me it was already a quiet place compared to the rest of Goa, but Stef told me that off-season Agonda was magically silent, apart from the sound of the high winds and battering rain. "It's so dramatic! It's wonderful!" he said.

During those first weeks, I shared breakfast time at Simrose with Sven from Germany who is still the happiest person I have ever met; he laughed like a drain at his own jokes. He told me he'd been mistaken for Bruce Willis by some Russians who asked for a selfie. Sven had an 'alpha' appearance – all muscles, tattoos, shaved head and earrings – but the faces of his two grown-up children were tattooed on his chest. He talked lovingly about his children and told me he had never touched a drop of alcohol. "Am I a real German?!" he cried, laughing. He told me he'd ordered a 'Sex on the Beach' cocktail the previous night, "without the alcohol and without the sex." We shared sobriety stories – I was coming up for my one-year 'soberversary'. I was encouraged by Sven's clear-eyed smile and sense of adventure.

Every day, Sven climbed onto his scooter and explored South Goa. I envied him his freedom. I was still too scared to ride a scooter, meaning my daily activities were restricted to Agonda unless I wanted to hire Mr Happy or a tuktuk. I decided on my second weekend in Agonda that I would go to the Saturday market in the nearest town, Chaudi, for a wander around. I asked Mr Happy to drive me there, as long as he promised to fix his brakes.

Chaudi market was the yellowest place I've ever visited, and therefore one of the happiest, filled with stallholders selling every kind of fruit, vegetable and spice, plus a range of plastic goods from combs to soap dishes. The main fruit and vegetable market was covered with huge yellow tarpaulins tied together, making the heaps of produce and the shoppers glow with good health. I didn't have a kitchen in the Red House so I didn't need anything, but I also didn't know what half the things were and was too shy to ask.

I walked down an alleyway lined with older women sitting cross-legged on mats selling fish and found a marigold garland seller, his stall draped with abundant flowers. In India, marigolds represent the sun, with their brightness and positive energy; Chaudi market was filled with sunshine that Saturday morning.

Like the magpie that I am, I found a young man selling sparkling beaded necklaces and bought three silvery ones to wear on the beach. I am drawn to bright, shining things, and I bought strands of tiny round mirrors to hang from my curtain rails at the Red House.

Back home, the mirrors sparkled in the sunlight next to my palm-tree-patterned curtains. I peeked through the window above my bed and saw the two pigs – whom I now called my 'chicas' – in the yard of the house behind mine. They were snuffling around, content in each other's company. I longed for Shubham to return.

Each working day, after breakfast with Sven in Simrose, I'd head to the other end of the village where Sampoorna Yoga School lay at the top of a red-dust track. I loved its warm-brown logo on the cream wall and the rainbow-coloured chalkboard next to it with its list of classes. The board stood at the entrance to the school opposite Mandala Café, owned by two brothers from Rajasthan: Ilu and Uday. Ilu was devastatingly good-looking with long, black hair tied in a man bun, an unbuttoned shirt, rolled-up jeans and layers of mala beads hanging over his bare chest (Shubham called this look 'rowdy style').

All the yoga girls (and boys) scurried into the café as Ilu 'arranged' his hair in the mirror at the back of the café each morning. It was a sight to behold. I'd smile at him in the mirror as I walked to work, and he'd wave back. He was a beautiful man who'd cause a frisson when he rode through Agonda on his Enfield, hair blowing in the wind – but underneath the peacocking, there was a man with kindness and humility.

What I loved about the café were the brightly coloured chairs and tables, the painted mandalas on the walls and the shrines to the gods and goddesses replete with marigold garlands. The boys played beautiful mantra music, and whilst they regularly chased cows out of the café with water spray, they also made sure the animals were fed and watered. They were kind as well as being devastatingly good-looking, which was the heady mix I'd fallen for in Shubham.

I shared an office at Sampoorna with some of the teachers and administration staff. Deepak and Eli, the owners of the school, showed me into the air-conditioned space and briefed me on what was needed. I was to write twenty-one blog posts on topics from why we say *namaste*, to the best yoga poses to beat the winter blues. I couldn't wait to get started. They allowed me to use the office for my other editorial work too.

I met Vijaya, a young Indian woman who was teaching anatomy on the week-long Yin Yoga course I'd be taking in December. Her head wobbled vigorously as she smiled and introduced herself, from behind a pile of anatomy books. It was her first teaching gig and she was creating the course manual from scratch.

Before lunch, I walked around the main Sampoorna shala and smiled, remembering my time as a student there only seven months previously; the sound of the staff chatting as they cleaned the huts, tended the jungle gardens and made the food. There were the jewelled cushions on the floor where my teachers Danni and Karen had sat, persuading me to stay and do the yoga teacher training, even though everything inside me was telling me I needed to go home.

Back then, I'd been full of self-doubt and fear. I didn't think I was good enough to train as a yoga teacher, but they said it wasn't about being good enough, it was about being self-aware and leaving my ego at the door. I tried to use the excuse of a shoulder injury. "Even better," they said. "Having an injury actually makes you even more aware of your body and your ego."

And even when I pushed through all of that, I was so afraid of not catching my flight back to the UK and choosing to stay another month. I was not a person who made decisions like that. I did not miss flights and I did not suddenly do something like stay in another country, let alone India, for a month.

Danni and Karen had interrogated me: "What are you going back for? A job?"

No. I was still freelance and no one was knocking my door down with another role on the corporate ladder. When I realised that the thing I was going back for was actually to get the roots of my hair done, I knew I had to stay. No more excuses.

"*Let your roots grow, Lisa,*" I thought. "*No one cares whether your hair is red or not except you.*"

So I stayed, I grew my silver hair and the whole experience changed my life. So much so, I wrote a book about it. But that book lay dormant in November 2019. I didn't know it, but there were still a few plot twists yet to be added to the story.

Every day, I'd roll out my mat after work and practice to the sound of the *poder*, back again at 5pm for the evening bread run, and the crows calling time on the day. Then the sunset would lure me back to the beach, not for a cocktail as it would have done in my former life, but to see Sanjo and Zimbo settling down for the evening in the sand, to see Nitesh pulling his boat back in, to wave at Dinesh as he bustled around families fitting in an early dinner with the kids, to be ignored by Sweetpea who was being fed by said kids, and to wave at Marshall who would be striding quickly down the beach with his friends, carrying a long stick.

I'd go back to Kopi Desa each evening, where I'd met Shubham in December 2017, and now longed for him to return. His friends, Shubham (there are lots of Shubhams in Goa) and Ram, treated me like a sister and I pulled up a bamboo stool while they plied me with lime and soda and hummus and pita bread.

And so began the routine of my days, happy writing and editing, happy to be back in the village I loved with the prospect of The Most Handsome Man in Goa's return. As the diggers retreated, old resorts rebuilt themselves (within the new constraints) and new shacks sprang up. Agonda's storm damage slowly cleared and blue skies returned after some intermittent post-monsoon rain showers. The dream I was supposed to be living was finally here.

One lunchtime at Sampoorna, Karen grabbed me as I was ladling various vegan dishes onto my metal *thali* plate. "I need an assistant!" she cried, wrapping the skein of her silken brown hair around her hand as her bright blue eyes flashed at me. Karen was a Canadian beauty, lightly tanned and freckled of skin with movie-star looks. I wasn't the only woman at the school with a yoga-goddess crush on her, especially when she swished into mealtimes wearing one of Gita's offerings. That day it was one of her cotton halterneck jumpsuits, elasticated around the ankles. I looked (and felt) a bit like a sexy Teletubby in mine, but Karen always managed to look like a creature of Rivendell.

"I think you could do it!" she continued. "I'd love it to be you... I mentioned it to Sudhir and he agreed I should ask you."

Sudhir, the director of the teacher-training courses at Sampoorna and the ex-monk who had changed my entire perspective on life with his yoga philosophy classes. Sudhir, the man with the widest, brightest smile of all smiles, the man whose mantra was and still is, '*Joy is my nature, smile is your birthright*'. He appeared as though we had manifested him behind Karen's shoulder, in his crisp, white, shortsleeved shirt and pressed slacks over his bare feet. "We need you, Lisa! We have been let down by someone in one of our teaching groups. Please think about joining us as a Karma Yogi for the rest of this term. It's only for a few weeks."

I felt overcome with emotion. I felt so honoured, so loved and so valued to be asked to be a Karma Yogi. These were coveted positions where yoga teachers gave their assistance in exchange for accommodation, food and classes. Their role was an act of service, in keeping with yoga philosophy. Karma Yoga is defined as the carrying out of action without any attachment to results, often more simply interpreted as 'selfless service'. The *Bhagavad Gita*, one of the best-known stories in Indian scripture, mentions it as one of the paths to spiritual liberation. *What better way to live the dream*, I thought.

I walked along the beach that evening with a full heart. I couldn't believe the Sampoorna staff had that much faith in me. I suddenly wondered if this was my calling. Was this what I was really meant to be doing after all? Was editing and writing just the sideshow and this the main perfor-mance? The emotion I'd felt at being asked was surely a sign that it was the right path – I always let myself be guided by my heart, rightly or wrongly.

As I walked back to the Red House, I passed a young British couple sitting on the sand, smiling at me. Behind me, I heard the young woman say to her partner, "It's so great to see someone truly happy." It took me a few seconds to realise that she meant me. I'd noticed people smiling at me a lot since my last visit to Goa, both in London and in India. I think I must have had a smile on my face without even real-ising it.

As I was already on the staff of Sampoorna, being a Karma Yogi (or KY) seemed like an easy segue, but I knew it would eat into my time. The KYs I'd encountered were ever-present and ever-available; their time not theirs – whatever they had to give belonged to the teachers and students. That was the point: selfless action with no regard for personal reward. My beloved mornings on the beach would go because I'd have to be ready to attend class at 6.30am, helping Karen with hands-on assists on the students. But I had a strong sense that the universe was moving me in this direction and decided to accept the role. I would fit my other work around it. It was only for a few weeks, after all.

The next morning, I walked along the beach road in the dark, hours before the *poder's* bicycle bell and Charlie's blue cart would open, with only a few snuffling cows and inquisitive dogs aware of my presence.

I slid into the shala at the back of Sampoorna, pushing through the muslin curtains designed to keep mosquitoes off, and received a small wave from Karen. The students were engaged in their silent mornings – no speaking until after morning classes were over – so I waved back. They were all waiting for the start of their '*Mysore*' Ashtanga practice – which meant they would guide themselves through the specific sequence of asanas (poses) at their own pace with visual prompts in front of them. Karen led them through the Ashtanga chant that opens every class – *Vande Gurunam...* – and then they began in silence.

I walked around the shala nervously assisting students, who were mostly young women in their twenties. There were grateful smiles and softly whispered questions. They were mostly keen for me to hold their legs in headstands at the end, I found, and appreciative of a head massage as they lay in *savasana*.

A couple of the girls came to talk to me after class, excited to hear my story, as someone who had already been through the training. I told them I'd only completed my training seven months before. That turned out to be a bad move.

The next time I attended the early morning class, a couple of the girls dismissed me when I came over to help. *Ok*, I thought – *not everyone needs help*. I remembered my own ego telling me I didn't need my KY's help when I was training. But then another student got annoyed with me because I couldn't answer her question and I began to worry that I wasn't experienced enough to help anyone. As the mornings went by, I let it affect my confidence. In the second week, my nervousness in the shala was palpable and it seemed to me that nobody wanted me there.

When the students were surveyed mid-course one of them said that she was unhappy that there was someone with so little training assisting in class (I wasn't the only teacher or assistant they complained about but it still hurt). In a matter of a week, I went from a confident fifty-two-year-old free-lance editor and writer living the dream by the Arabian Sea, to someone fighting back tears in a yoga studio full of young women.

I talked to Karen about it one lunchtime and she said that people tended to bring all their fears and insecurities to the shala, and sometimes those fears and insecurities got directed at the teacher. But my own fears and insecurities appeared to be the problem now. I felt like a failure. I'd been given this huge opportunity and I feared that I simply couldn't cut it. I was a relative newbie trying to pass myself off as a fully fledged yogi. I was an imposter.

I began to dread every morning class and missed my sunrise walks terribly. In the afternoons I'd been drafted in to help Karen assess all the students' teaching practice but the blow to my confidence affected my ability to be helpful in any meaningful way. Plus, my one attempt at being authoritative had backfired.

Karen gave me the chance to address the group at the start of one of the teaching sessions and I told the students that creating a great class wasn't about them, it was about their students' experience. '*It's not about you*' was the kind of thing I'd have said to my old publishing team back in London but afterwards, Karen took me to one side and said I'd been too harsh, that the teaching at Sampoorna worked on positive reinforcement.

I was confused because the one thing I'd learned was that yoga was about service to others, which meant it was never about oneself. I was shocked by the negative feedback, especially as I'd prided myself on managing people very effectively. It was my 'thing', but yoga seemed to be intent on pulling everything I once thought about myself apart and forcing me to assess each piece, as I'd done with the contents of my home, before deciding to keep it or throw it out.

The next day, I was sharing more of my concerns with Karen in the dining area. Sudhir came over and asked us why we were both frowning; he didn't like it if we were less than openly happy in front of the students. But I couldn't pretend to be happy if I wasn't and I'd found the whole yogic concept of conscious cheerfulness – *santosha* – the most difficult to master. I knew that the other teachers and Karma Yogis were much better at it than me, and I knew that I was bringing the vibe down. But I couldn't seem to help it.

Misery loves company and as I shared my woes with Vijaya day after day in the office I could see that I was bringing her down too. I didn't know what to do with the tidal wave of emotions I was dealing with. I was programmed to share everything with everyone and didn't know how to process it all myself.

One morning, when I wasn't at Sampoorna, I took my regular walk to the place where the ocean met the river at the end of the beach. I tried to work out why I wasn't more grateful for my new role and why it was making me so unhappy. This was Sampoorna, one of the most prestigious yoga schools in the world! I felt guilty at the thought of walking away from it – I was being given an opportunity others would give anything for. But I felt like I hadn't earned my place there. I felt like a fraud, trying to pass off my seven months' experience as seven years to a group of young women. After twenty-five years of experience in another industry that had got me to a coveted top spot, I was back on the first rung of the ladder again.

And then there was the group itself. One young woman had attached herself to me early on – she was friendly and filled with questions at first. But as time went on, she was one of students who batted me away if I tried to help her. She seemed to be the ringleader of a small group of girls who all began to react to me in the same way.

But I was not, I decided, going to allow myself to go from high-powered manager to being battered by the emotional baggage of a group of 'mean girls' at the age of fifty-two. I'd have had children if I was up for that in any way. When it came to the group's closing ceremony – a *puja* or fire ceremony where all the graduates wore white – I didn't go. I didn't even consider it as an option – I was only a temporary replacement anyway, not a true part of the teaching team.

Word came the next day that Sudhir was upset that I hadn't turned up at the ceremony, and that the girls in the class I'd assisted had got me a card and a present. Karen saw

me at Kopi Desa that same night and handed me their card
and a tiny package containing a necklace. I immediately felt
guilty and wondered if I'd been wrong about the mean girls.
But when I opened the card back at the Red House the
message stung: *"Dear Lisa. It was such a pleasure to witness
your growth on your journey with us."* I felt insulted and
patronised and vowed never to put myself in that position
again. I was so angry that I threw the necklace in the bin
immediately.

The next day, I spoke to Sudhir and Karen and said that
being a Karma Yogi wasn't for me. It was making me miserable and I wanted to go back to just writing blogs for the
school. At least with writing I felt confident and fluent. No
mean girls could take that away from me. They agreed to let
me go.

I started my Yin Yoga training the following week,
learning about its emphasis on slowness and stillness as a way
to make the body release any tension it was holding onto. It
worked with the Chinese system of 'meridians' – energy
channels that control balance in the body in the way that the
Indian 'nadis' are said to do. (Both meridians and nadis line
up with the major systems of the body expressed in Western
medicine, for example, the nervous or circulatory systems.)

I'd discovered during my initial teacher-training that
there was a reason why my own shoulders and hips had been
so painful for a number of years: they were points in the body
that absorbed stress, where the body curled inwards, foetally,
to defend itself. Yoga was the process of uncurling and
releasing stress. It had led me to a place where I had been
able to face the world without the aid of alcohol, to see my
working life as the unnecessary stressor that it was and to
look life in the eye clearly, with nothing to blur the view.

I began to value Yin's slowness, with a lack of performance that I'd seen in other forms of yoga. I wondered if it was more my thing – it was definitely more in tune with my body which was criss-crossed by knots of fascia and muscle, built up over decades of tension. Sitting in each pose for at least three minutes stopped me in my tracks and allowed me to breathe. But what I didn't expect was that it would continue to release a torrent of unexpected emotions.

The group – all women, mostly over thirty – were experienced yoga practitioners and teachers. We bonded in Sampoorna's bright shalas but it became evident that what some of us were bonding over was being highly critical of the course, the teachers and each other. I'd left behind post-work bitching sessions in the pub with my old corporate life, but here they were again, those spiralling negative discussions, and I was a willing participant.

One day, before the exam at end of the course, I decided not to socialise with the group anymore. It was as much to protect them from me as it was myself from them. I could see that we were all in an unhealthy dynamic, bringing all our fears and insecurities from our non-yoga lives into the shalas. We were the mean girls, all grown up. I knew I was bringing my own ego into the shala and the school office and inflicting its agonised thrashings on everyone around me, because I didn't know where else to take my emotions.

In the cold light of sober days, I wondered why I was so highly critical of everything. I'd actually spoilt my teacher graduation ceremony in May 2019 because of it. I'd had a wonderful young teacher in the drop-ins who became one of my teachers on the course and I was delighted to be in her group. She was inexperienced, as I had been as a KY, but Sudhir had seen her potential and given her an opportunity.

But it was clear as the course went on that the other group were getting a different level of teaching to ours and my ego began to demand the same for me. I let that ego complain to Sudhir and he had taken her to one side and fed back the information. Things didn't improve, so when it came to the final student survey, I felt I had no choice but to leave a complaint again, as nicely worded as I could. What I hadn't bargained on was my complaint not being the only one and the feedback being given to the teacher right before the graduation ceremony.

At an event that is meant to be a joyful moment after four weeks of intense training, I felt wretched. I could see the effect it had had on that young teacher and how another teacher had held her hand throughout the ceremony. She was clearly close to tears.

As we trooped down to the beach, all in white and garlanded in marigolds for our photo session, I couldn't muster the energy or smiles to join in with the festivities. Instead, I posed with my friend Chris for a few photos and walked down to Simrose to see the dogs instead. My overriding memory of that day was of sitting in between Sanjo and Zimbo on the sand, feeling so sad that I'd upset that teacher and spoilt both of our experiences.

When the Yin training ended, everyone in the group was handed a survey and back at the Red House, I began to fill it in with all my recommendations for improving it. It was the editor in me at work, but it was also the ego in me. I questioned what I was doing.

Why did I feel such an intense desire to critique everything and everyone? It was something that was useful in my work as an editor and manager but this wasn't confined to my working life. Why was I still so keen to pull other things to shreds – not just books, but people and the work they were doing? Why was I so angry about everything and with everyone, still, after all the yoga training, the therapy, the giving up of alcohol and the discovery of Little Lisa? Who was I really angry with?

Much later, I realised that my ego had been the one to accept the Karma Yogi role (so much for selfless acts), it was my ego that was so hurt by the students' comments and it was my ego that insisted on blaming everyone and everything around it. But the person I was really blaming for everything was me.

I ripped up the pages of the survey and threw them in the bin. And thank goodness, because at that graduation ceremony, Deepak and Eli made the most beautiful speech about me, grateful to their 'writer-in-residence'. I was deeply humbled and learned a lesson in gratitude.

'*Stop focusing on what is wrong with everything*,' I thought, making a new life rule for myself. '*Focus on what is right and be grateful for everything you can learn from it.*'

Despite my failure at Karma Yogi-ship, Karen was still pushing for me to take on teaching work at Sampoorna and put my name down to teach drop-in classes in the main shala. My ego and confidence had taken a beating, but at least the classes would be in the late afternoons so I could regain my morning walks and the people in the classes would be different each day. I would start with a 'gentle vinyasa' 4pm class which I knew from experience only attracted a handful of people who didn't want an energetic workout. That was what the morning classes were for.

Then a week later in early December, a bomb dropped. The 9.30am drop-in class teacher was ill and I was asked to stand in for them. It was a vinyasa class and those that turned up for it would be expecting a certain calibre of teacher, someone who could perform the asana 'greats' of yoga.

Karen was super-supportive as usual over a smoothie bowl in Mandala café. "I'll come along! I'll be there at the back!" she said encouragingly.

"Please don't!" I shouted, filled with horror. The last thing I needed was a yoga goddess at the back of my class, giving me feedback at the end. Sure, I could give out criticism, but could I take it myself? No, I could not.

The day before the class was spent learning my sequence off by heart so that I could concentrate on the teaching of it. I wrote it all out neatly in a new leather-bound book I bought at Gita's stall. Vinyasa is a bit like dancing, the poses flowing from one to another, so I was taken swiftly back to my years of ballet teaching. Surely that would stand me in good stead?

That night I barely slept and I couldn't face any food. All I kept thinking was that in a few hours' time, it would be over. I would have taught my first serious class at Sampoorna Yoga School. Even though I was a seven-month-only fraud.

Primed with my ninety-minute soundtrack, savasana oils and notebook, I arrived early at the shala and set up my speaker and mat at the front of the room. Slowly, students began to arrive and I tried not to see disappointment on their faces when they realised I was teaching and not their favourite goddess. But somehow I got through the class and only a couple of the thirty or so people left during it. This was fairly commonplace – I'd left classes myself for various reasons so I tried not to take it personally.

Afterwards, I threw myself onto the jewelled cushions in

the restaurant, relieved to be joining all the other teachers for breakfast.

"Nice class," a voice said.

It was Nadja, a German teacher whom I'd noticed adding 'extras' to my sequences to get more of a workout in. I knew I'd be too gentle and slow for some people and I'd prepared myself for it. At least she hadn't left early.

"It was a really good basic vinyasa class. I really must try and get back to that myself. I always make everything too complicated."

Basic. It was a bell that clanged in my head. I had taught a *basic* yoga class. Yet again, I was an imposter, masquerading as something I wasn't: a good yoga teacher.

If I heard that now, I'd take it as a compliment – I know some teachers embellish their sequences to the point where some students can't keep up or feel inferior because their bodies can't 'perform' the sequences. But back then I shuddered. I knew I'd delivered a 'good enough' class but maybe the people that left did so because they weren't getting their workout for the day. If my name was on the roster again, they'd be rolling their eyes and swerving the shala altogether.

But then, as I walked past Mandala on my way home, another voice spoke quietly to me. "Thank you for a lovely class."

It was a tall, blonde, crop-haired teacher from a nearby school. I'd seen her come in just as I was about to start teaching and my stomach had lurched in fear. Grateful for her feedback, I told her how nervous I'd been.

"There is always something you can learn, no matter who is teaching, or what is taught. You can learn about your response to it."

If only every teacher thought as she did, I thought.

If only I could think like that.

I got back to the Red House and walked through the garden towards the white tiled steps up to my room. I'd washed and hung up my clothes to dry that morning but now there was something very obviously missing on the line. I looked at all the yoga leggings and bra tops and dresses and couldn't see my new green snakeskin leggings. Gita found them hilarious: "You look like a snake!" she'd said, the first time I wore them. I immediately thought someone had stolen them.

Suddenly, Marshall my landlord ran round the corner, brandishing his beach cane: "It's a cow! He stole my daughter's things!"

We ran down the road together and there, in front of the church, were my green leggings squished into the road, the backs of several cows retreating into the distance. All the tuktuk drivers sitting on the church steps shouted in unison, "It was a cow! She has your clothes!"

"Thanks for retrieving them, guys!" I shouted as they grinned at me, unmoving, watching me shake my leggings out of the dust.

Needless to say, I asked my landlady, Saluzhina, to start doing my washing. After the first load I asked her what I should pay and Marshall said, "Pay what you think is right."

I offered 400 rupees (roughly £4) but it was obviously wrong because neither of them answered me. That afternoon, I checked the going rate in a few shops and it turned out to be around 200 rupees, which I went back and offered.

"Too much – 150," Saluzhina replied, giving me my change.

"And what?"

There he was, The Most Handsome Man in Goa, my Shubham, wearing a *'Wilder Than You Think'* T-shirt. He was one of the gentlest men I'd ever met, standing tall and broad-shouldered, his hair in loose black curls. His colleagues and regulars nicknamed him 'Shaggy'.

"What is this wild side you've never told me about, Shub?" I asked, grinning. "Are you a bit of a dark horse?"

"I have many dark horses," he replied, his thick black eyebrows settling into a humorous frown.

We always joked about the fact that his sexy frown made me think he was a player; a ladykiller who worked the bars of Agonda and had a different woman in every port. His frown was and is the facial expression of movie stars, a real Blue Steel, making the most of his beautiful Goan eyes. In reality, that frown was simply his concentration face, the one he adopted when he made cocktails at Kopi Desa. In his heart, Shubham was a man who tended a garden and made toys for his nephew out of shells and driftwood. He had a stammer that got worse when he was stressed, which was almost never.

It was the first week in December and we'd been messaging constantly, whenever he was in port, because we hadn't seen each other for nine months. We had fantasised about this moment of meeting again, whilst retelling the story of how we met over and over. It was a story we never tired of.

I returned to the bar that night, dressed to the nines in a top from Gita's newest collection: an aquamarine silk halter-neck in a paisley pattern, paired with my silver bias-cut long skirt and silver sandals. I wanted to look good for my man. My dark horse.

But I still had my reservations. Not only was this man

half my age but so far it was just an extended holiday romance where both parties had only been in the same room together for less than three months. I felt sure that there was more to our relationship than that, but me living here for a while would give me the answers I needed.

I had my independence and freedom in the Red House and my work and friends at Sampoorna and Simrose. I wanted to protect that freedom but explore the joy of being with someone who had made my heart flood with love. *'Tis better to have loved and lost, than never to have loved at all*, I told myself, quoting Tennyson.

We carried on where we'd left off the previous April – Shubham taking me out for rides on his bike to remote beaches and then early dinner afterwards. He took me north to Canaguinim, where a small river met the sea and a few brightly coloured villas sat within a cluster of palm trees behind an empty golden beach. Someone had made a heart in the sand out of upturned beer bottles.

We fantasised about living here, this mini Agonda, and Shubham opening '*Shaggy's Shack*' where he'd serve cock-tails (and mocktails for me). There was an empty villa, an intense turquoise blue with white paintwork, where I imag-ined waking up and walking down to the beach at dawn, my hand in Shubham's, as the local dogs stretched on the sand.

On the way back, the sun lowering in the sky, we'd take the winding road to Cabo de Rama fort, its red stones glowing in the late afternoon heat. Golden-furred langur monkeys would swing through the trees around us, babies on their backs, looking for their evening meal. Shubham insisted on taking pictures of me at one of the viewing platforms over-looking the sea. It was something I loved about him – after a marriage where I'd had to ask for my photo to be taken if I wanted one as a keepsake, it was so nice to have someone say, "Let me click a picture of you. Stand over there!"

Shubham would be working at Kopi in the evenings so we'd stop for an early dinner at Red Crab restaurant nearby as the sun set. Wicker tables and chairs were set out on a small platform right on the edge of the coastline, where a dizzying, dazzling view of swaying palms and glittering ocean accompanied our Goan fish suppers.

This routine was a dream that had kept me going through our time apart and it was just as beautiful, even more so, than I'd remembered. The best part was holding on to Shubham as dusk fell across the winding roads back to Agonda, where the evening lights shimmered like a strand of crystal beads.

We'd pass the 'bat tree' which was filled with screeching fruit bats, flexing their wings and conducting test flights over our heads. We'd get stuck in a traffic jam that would turn out to be a cow refusing to get out of the way, but it would give me time to observe people making small fires outside their shops or laughing with friends outside the temple.

As we sped by, I liked looking inside the shops filled with Kashmiri shawls and mirrored lamps and finding Zimbo and Sanjo in their evening resting place – outside their owner's shop beside the back entrance to Simrose. Women had water bottles filled with a golden liquid standing outside their clothing stalls: petrol top-ups for those caught short on their bikes and tuktuks.

The dream of being reunited had become a reality, but it also quickly became apparent that wasn't going to happen very much. Shubham's first priority on his return was of course, his family. His parents, four sisters and a nephew were all used to seeing him every day, but they'd lost him to the ocean for the previous nine months. They didn't know about me, waiting in the Red House for my love, and I knew that if they did, they might not be very happy.

Shubham's days were busy so I often got the convenient evening slot while he was working at the bar in Agonda and his family and friends in Palolem and Patnem were given the daylight hours. I knew that it was a logical outcome of his work schedule and geographical location but inside, I felt like I was becoming Nighttime Girlfriend and every ounce of me railed against it.

Before Shubham, I'd 'dated' an Algerian man for two years who'd made me his Nighttime Girlfriend, only coming round to my flat in London for some 'girlfriend experience' time which amounted to watching the TV, sex, sleeping over and coffee in bed. The rest of his time was devoted to work and his friends. And now, I felt like the same thing was starting to happen, albeit for a different reason.

Night after night, I'd dress up for my 'date' with Shubham as he worked behind the bar and at closing time, he would come to the Red House to see me. Eventually, I explained my concerns about becoming Nighttime Girl-friend and Shubham's frown appeared. But this time, it meant that he was cross.

"You think I want you only for one thing?" he said, aghast. "Is that what you think?!"

"No, I know you don't. It's just I—"

"I am not like those men before. I just want to see you. I want to be with you."

Shubham explained that he had responsibilities to his family in the morning, friends in the afternoon and it was more convenient to see me in the evenings and overnight because he'd be in Agonda anyway. I got it. But it played into my fear of being kept in the dark and hidden away.

Above everything, I wanted to walk in the daylight hand-in-hand with someone and not be their secret. I knew that Shubham felt torn between his traditional family life, his friends and me. I was the odd-one-out in that triangle, the one that couldn't easily be fitted in anywhere. It helped that our adventures played out in another town to the one he lived in, at the end of every day. But it began to make me feel sad.

So, when it came to closing time, I started to say no. I wanted to sleep, especially now that I wasn't trying to get drunk every evening, and I wanted to get up early and walk on the beach. I knew that Shubham's schedule was go to bed late, sleep late, see family and friends, go to work and I refused to take the nightshift. I was too old for that, for one thing.

And so, it transpired that Shubham and I would only manage a whole day together every two weeks, because of my insistence on being Daytime Girlfriend. But they were perfect days. They were made of sparkling seas and splashing in the water, Shubham holding me safe in the rough waves, his oiled hair gleaming like a seal's.

I would cling to his sides on the back of the Enfield, trying not to squeeze too hard as we rode around bends and making sure I leaned the same way. I was terrified of falling off and sang mantras to distract myself. Shubham would laugh at my 'scary' and rub my leg affectionately.

Those days, although few and far between, were like the small round mirrors hanging in my room at the Red House. They flashed white with sunlight and temporary blinded me to reality. In my heart, I knew that what I had with Shubham might only happen in those moments, so I cherished every glittering scene as though it were the last.

In the weeks leading up to Christmas, I realised that the thing most affecting our daytime moments was Shubham's partying, which was entirely normal for a twenty-five-year-old. I didn't want to be around anyone who was drinking, which meant he'd go to parties without me. When he *was* free, he'd ask if I wanted to see him that night and I'd say no. We went round and round on the same carousel for weeks and I started to realise we were leading two separate lives, largely down to our age difference and me being sober. I couldn't be the one to stop him partying and he couldn't be the one to tempt me back into drinking.

I had made friends with Sally at this point – she was the British girlfriend of the Indian man who ran Love Bites, the unfortunately named café behind the Red House. Its name belied the fact that it was a wonderful, cosy place with great North Indian food – the owner, Rahul, hailed from Shimla in Himachal Pradesh.

The café was on two floors; downstairs had gaily painted chairs and tables while the upstairs – which was a rather wobbly plinth made from strapped wooden poles and planks – was scattered with cushions and mats and low tables. Of course it was this high place that I loved, especially during hot afternoons when I could lie down and let the cool breeze coming off the sea wash over me. I could also get a superb smoothie bowl – a breakfast staple in Agonda – filled with fruit, seeds and nuts. I had mine with coffee and toast on the side.

I told Sally about my predicament and she knew exactly what I was talking about. "It's not easy dating an Indian man," she told me. "There is an expectation that you'll fit in with their lives at some point, even if what attracted them to you at a certain point was your independence and freedom."

To me it sounded like any man's expectation. It reminded me of a conversation I'd had with a friend back home in the UK some years before. She was extremely gregarious and sociable and loved to dance. She'd dated a man who'd loved all those things about her when they met, but then slowly objected to everything, including her dancing. Shubham wasn't stopping me dancing, but there was clearly nowhere where I could join him on his dance floor.

Most afternoons I'd sit in my Red House room, working and practising yoga, hoping that Shubham would rock up on his bike to surprise me but he didn't.

But my disappointment was mixed with an unexpected sort of relief – I wanted to get on with my new life and work routine but at the same time I wanted it all to be interrupted by this inconvenient wonderful young man.

By the same token, I wondered if Shubham wanted to be with his family and friends and at the same time be interrupted by an inconvenient wonderful older woman.

I was hoping we could find a way to meet in the middle.

Finally, Christmas arrived, and I'd been invited to festivities at the Red House, by Marshall, Saluzhina and their daughter, Bethany, who were all Catholics. I decided to start the day by attending mass at the local church even though I was no longer a believer. Going into Catholic churches when I was abroad was something I did to honour the memory of my mother. I liked to light candles for her.

Christmas in Goa is a glorious affair with lit paper stars

of all colours festooning the houses. The day before Christmas Eve, I visited the churches and the cathedrals of Old Goa, further north. It was like a theme park devoted to the Holy Family, and every church had its own flashing nativity scene with a recumbent Baby Jesus as the star of the show. I found it weird that so much devotion was being shown by Indian families to such a blazingly white, blond baby.

Like many Goan churches, St Anne's in Agonda is a huge, white, iced wedding cake of a building. On Christmas morning it was festooned with a pink blousy canopy out front to shade the overspilled congregation (and the various tuktuk drivers waiting for business and watching cows trample yoga leggings).

On Christmas morning, the service itself was fairly generic but during Holy Communion, I noticed a Western woman having trouble walking down the aisle to the priest. She was crying her eyes out and I wanted to give her a hug. I think I needed one too, when I saw the priest speak kindly to her and offer her words of comfort.

Something about Christmas always got to me – the memories of family Christmasses past, and how there would never be another. My father died of bowel cancer when I was ten and my mother from a heart attack (she had dementia) when I was thirty-two. Twenty years later and the grief hadn't left me; it came in unexpected waves at times like this.

After mass, I turned up to Marshall's door having bought a painted-glass candlestick as a gift, which I immediately broke by hitting it on the stair rail. Oh well – it was the thought that counted. Marshall told me that his family didn't exchange gifts at Christmas – the red ones under his tree were fake. The real gifts were offering food and opening your house to family and friends; presence, not presents.

Inside, we all gathered, shepherd-like, around Elish, Marshall's grandson. He was a smiling, gurgling, laughing boy who wore black and white bangles around his little wrists and black kohl around his eyes to protect against evil spirits. They made him look even more beautiful than he already was.

Marshall and Saluzhina guided me into a room where all the food was beautifully laid out – curries of every kind – and I spooned them onto a bed of rice on my plate. I'd told Marshall that I was vegetarian, but somehow all the dishes contained chicken and I didn't have the heart to refuse them.

When I returned to my room and looked out of my window, there was only one chica to be seen. I hoped beyond hope that her partner hadn't gone into one of the curries.

———

After Christmas, Shubham took me on the Enfield to Galgibaga, a turtle-nesting beach like the one at Agonda but bigger and emptier. It was lined with casuarina trees, not palms, affording shade from the blistering heat. We played in the sea, then threw ourselves on patterned cotton throws under the trees to dry out.

"This is how I want our time together to be spent," I told him, turning on my side to face him. "In full daylight."

"I know, babe, but I have things to do – for my family – and my friends want to see me too, before I go back on ship. I have to look after my nephew..."

"I've worked out that we've only seen each other like this

one time every two weeks," I stated boldly. I knew that
Shubham responded to statements with numbers in them.

"I'm sorry, babe. I don't know what to do."

I knew it was difficult for Shubham to balance the expectations of his family and his friends, who were begging him to
hang out with them every day. Perhaps it was unfair of me to
expect him to apportion to time to me, especially as we
weren't 'official' and he was having to hide my existence from
his family. I had some serious thinking to do.

As New Year approached – the two-year anniversary of
Shubham and me getting together approached and my reso-
lutions had formed. I decided to say a firm 'no' to the darkness of Nighttime Girlfriend forever and 'yes' to the daylight.
I would not compromise my early morning walks with the
pack and the sunrise for some snatched hours with Shubham
at night. I'd compromised myself in this way for nine years
after I left my husband and that phase, I decided, was over.

This had been more than a holiday romance, but it was a
no-mans-land that I couldn't stay in. I wanted clarity. We
were not in an official relationship and I would confirm that
as soon as I could with Shubham. I would tell him that I was
hanging on in a sort of limbo and I needed to be let go, to be
free again. In exchange, Shubham could live his own life and
pursue his own future. We could still see each other, but
with no expectations on either side. It would be easier
that way.

As if he knew what I was about to say, Shubham
suddenly disappeared for three days without telling me. I
discovered that he'd gone to the Sunburn music festival in

North Goa with his friends and it was likely that he was going crazy, because he could without me there to kill his vibe. I decided that this was a sign that we were completely over and this was his way of letting me know. Angry with myself and with him for disappearing, I put all the things he'd left in my room in a small plastic bag and delivered it to the boys at Kopi Desa.

When I arrived at the bar, Ram looked scared.

"This is for Shubham," I barked angrily.

"He's... He's... not here," Ram said quietly, looking over his shoulder as Shubham the bar manager approached.

"I know he's not here, that's why I'm giving this to you," I shouted. I was breathing heavily.

"But it might get stolen here..." they both said, their voices trailing off.

"Well, that's not my problem," I replied, and stomped back to the Red House.

This wasn't the first time a red mist had descended in recent months. Whether I was in the yoga school or working on my laptop at Simrose, I'd found myself getting irrationally angry over the smallest things and angry with some of the people I was working with back in the UK. I had no control over it and words I knew I shouldn't say would spill out in emails or voice calls. I'd put it down to the stress of being in another country and away from 'normality', whatever that was. I'd got so emotional over the mean-girl situation at Sampoorna too, and I was someone who largely had their emotions under control.

Years before, a young man in publishing had accused me

of '*age-related crankiness*' as a joke. The words pinged back
into my mind as I walked back from Kopi Desa having left
Shubham's things with Ram. Was my crankiness age-related?
Or was something else at play? On one of my bad days, a
perceptive yoga teacher at Sampoorna said that I was clearly
being affected by the full moon. I hadn't even thought about
it before, but I realised that yes, I was feeling emotionally
overwrought at the same time at that month's full moon. I
began to track my moods with the lunar cycle to see if she
was right.

In a bid to arrest my emotional state and to stop me
thinking about Shubham, I threw myself into my self-prac-
tice yoga, having been told by the same teacher that solo
yoga, not group class, was the real deal. I also began swimming at my Secret Swimming Location. Marshall's niece
worked at a boutique resort in the village, down a track opposite Kopi Desa, where she would let me use the tiny pool for
free. I'd only learned to swim the previous year, so the sea
was too rough for me. At least there I could keep my practice
going in the most sublime surroundings.

As I backstroked up and down the pool, I watched the
crows, bats and sea eagles flit and soar overhead between the
palms and muffled their sounds out as the water covered my
ears. The heat of dry-season Agonda had got to me, but here I
could find a temperature that suited my body and calmed my
hot-headed emotions. Why was I responding so angrily to
everything, when clearly I was living in an earthly paradise?
They were stupid things to be angry about too – apart from
Shubham's disappearance – and I'd always been calm in my
work. Or had I? My last couple of years as a publishing
director in a toxic environment had led me to uncontrolled
outbursts both in emails and in person. One of my male

bosses had taken me to one side and said that although I was making very valid points, all people would remember would be my outbursts, not the points I was trying to make.

After the Sunburn festival was over, Shubham reappeared at the bar, just as usual, frowning over the cocktails he was making. When he first saw me, he seemed apologetic and humbled, but, as I socialised happily in front of him with the other 'Britishers' at the bar, he looked furious. I had turned the switch off on our 'relationship' without even having to say a word and he seemed to know what I'd done, simply from receiving his bag of belongings. And he clearly hated it. He spent several evenings glaring at me under his steeply angled brows.

Part of me wanted to be able to let him go, to see him fly through life with someone his own age, but part of me knew I'd be devastated to see it happen. I knew I'd have to cut off all contact with him if I did and I wasn't sure if I was ready for that. I still looked forward to seeing him at the bar every night, even when he was glaring at me. At least we were making eye contact.

New Year's Eve approached and I felt sad because the memory of my first big moment with Shubham was still fresh from two years before. We'd gone over and over the events of that sparkling night in our video calls, from the party I'd attended at my friend Guru's house, with its balcony overlooking the lights of Agonda, to the moment Shubham found me on the beach after midnight, with a bottle of sparkling wine and two glasses in his pack. We'd ridden on his Enfield back to Simrose where I was staying in a beachside hut and found ourselves unable to stop looking into each other's souls the next morning.

I was planning to attend the same beach party this year, but this time with friends from the bar, mainly British tourists who were staying for the season. Even though I was sober, I found myself socialising with a huge group of drinkers, who partied all night, slept until noon and started it all over again at lunchtime. They were great people – especially a couple I'd befriended who quickly became the centre of the social scene.

Hannah and Dave hailed from Kent and they were the opposite of me and Shubham: she was as young to Dave as Shubham was to me. Age-gap relationships appeared to be a thing among the travel community in this part of India where anything went, but of course here, as back at home, the only socially condoned age-gaps were ones where the man was older than the woman. No one blinked an eye over Hannah and Dave, but I was called a 'cougar' by other Brits, who sidled up to me at the bar to raise their eyebrows and make their point.

But this wasn't an unusual scenario for me – I'd been dating younger men ever since I left my marriage. To me, the idea of a predatory cougar was a complete myth – it was always the boys that made the first move (and then pretended I was chasing them). It was one of the great delights of my forties – discovering this unheralded new horizon of dating. No one told me that younger men would be waiting in the wings to meet me for the surge of sexuality I'd experience in my forties, a last hurrah for my ovaries. When I met Shubham, I thought I'd left that phase of my life behind, but clearly it was now an established pattern.

The plan was for the three of us – Hannah, Dave and I –

to head to H2o resort as soon as Kopi closed for the night. I was wondering where the bar staff would go to party – probably somewhere in Palolem where Shubham lived. It was a bigger town with more bars, clubs and restaurants – somewhere I didn't fancy at all.

I was sober so I knew I wouldn't be crying in the toilets over Shubham, the way I would have done when I used to binge-drink only a year previously. My drinking had started as a way to numb the pain of losing my parents but had gained pace with a stressful job in publishing and an unhappy marriage to a man who didn't love me. But, with the help of good therapy, the yoga course at Sampoorna and the people I'd encountered in Agonda, I'd managed to kick it. For me, New Year was time to celebrate in a different way.

At this stage I was still enjoying being the sober one while others got trashed – at least I could walk away and go back to my room at the Red House once I'd had enough. I couldn't believe that I'd once been the same as them – telling someone the same story over and over again. I suppose if you're only telling other drunk people, they don't notice. I'd been doing that only a year ago, propping up the bar at Kopi and slurring a few drinks later. I thought that was real life, until I realised it was slowly robbing me of mine.

Back in 2018, a friend from my hiking group said she was coming to spend Christmas in Agonda at the same time as me. She was great fun – we'd been drinking buddies on many hikes, when we were scouting around for allies and found each other. (I forged so many friendships over post-hiking boozing, but I also ended up spoiling a few too.)

At first, when Kim told me she was coming, I pictured us both staggering around the town and along the beach, going from bar to bar on Christmas Day, having as much fun as you could have at our age. But as the date grew closer, I had started thinking about giving up drinking and I knew I didn't want to spend Christmas with a huge hangover. I knew her expectation would be a drinking holiday and I was about to disappoint her. But then she landed in Goa ... and I heard nothing.

A day or so passed and I waited for a text, and finally received one from the resort she was staying at – it was at the other end of the beach, the sister resort to Simrose. We arranged to meet at Simrose to have dinner, drinks and a good old chat.

When she arrived, Kim told me that she'd spent the last two days in her hut, mainly drinking with the boys at the resort bar. *Fair enough*, I thought – I'd stayed in Simrose for three days when I first arrived in India and found solace in evening cocktails (although the 'boys' weren't allowed to drink with me).

We met for Christmas dinner at Kopi Desa and afterwards, I expected to see Kim on a couple of nights more, maybe for a few more drinks, but she went quiet again. I'd go to bed at 10pm and wake up to some drunken texts from her, including blurred images of vodka bottles next to her beach towel. Booze was very cheap at the local off-licence – I'd got my last bottle of sparkling wine there a year ago. She told me she'd shared the bottles with the resort staff and showed off to me about having a 'lock-in' there.

I started avoiding the end of the beach where she was staying, up near the river, normally my special place where I went for deep contemplation. But it felt like a black cloud was sitting above it and I couldn't bear to be near it. I dreaded getting a text or call from her, asking to meet up, but in fact, Kim was happily spending the whole of her time in

Agonda drinking in her hut. I knew she'd come out of an unhappy marriage with a man who was addicted to gambling and now I could see that his addiction had led to hers.

On her final morning, I received another text from her in the early hours, telling me to do exactly what I was already doing, which was to stay in India and enjoy getting to know the locals and travel around. I was furious! Who was she to tell me what I should be doing here, when she had been the one to copy my holiday?!

The denouement came when she left that night without seeing me. The next day, she posted all my morning beach photos on her own Facebook page, with her bottle photos interspersed among them. She wrote: *"Have had a wonderful time in India. I'll be back!"*

I commented straightaway: *"Images copyright: Lisa Edwards [winky face emoji]"*

"Sue me," she said with a winky face emoji back. She was a lawyer.

I knew that people came to Agonda to escape their real lives and live a fantasy one for a while. Hell, that's exactly what I'd been doing. But the reality was that their (and my) dark horses waited for them on the shore of this paradise beach and made them drink even more to try and drown them for good.

Back in Agonda in December 2019 and sober, I could see very clearly my own behaviour reflected in those that hadn't yet found a way to vanquish their demons. It served as a daily reminder to me that I could never let them win again. I had to stay strong.

And so, on New Year's Eve, I stood on the sand with my friends, Hannah and Dave, watching the fireworks, sober. I'd stayed up far longer than usual – midnight! – and was already planning my escape to the Red House. French exits – where one slipped away unannounced while no one was looking – had become my forte by this point and I was just about to do one when Shubham appeared.

I tried to control my delight as he approached me on the sand, just like he had two years ago. "Well, hello you. This reminds me of another time. You are in exactly the same place with exactly the same smile at exactly the same time."

"I know. I have that type of talent," Shubham said, grinning. "Can we go for a walk?"

I left Hannah and Dave and walked along the dark beach with Shubham, gazing at the phosphorescent waves. I didn't rush back into his arms, but I let him hold my hand.

"I'm sorry. I have been feeling a bit of crazy," he began. "I missed you, my Lisa."

"You could have messaged to say where you were going?" I said, biting back my annoyance. 'You disappeared for three days and then looked at me like I'd done something terrible!"

"I'm sorry. It's my volcano inside. It bubbles up sometimes and makes me angry."

As we walked in silence along the beach, fireworks bursting above our heads, I knew that Shubham's 'crazy' was struggling to make sense of a world of family, friendship and me and I refused to tell him off for his behaviour, to be 'mother'.

I also knew, because I'd had young boyfriends before, that Shubham was doing what twentysomethings do – asserting his freedom and independence and running away from situations with too much emotional pressure. My heart softened with his apology and we became friends again.

RAJASTHAN

I HAD ALREADY PLANNED TO VISIT THE JAIPUR Literature Festival at the end of January. It would be my first trip outside Goa and it was to a free public event attended by 400,000 people. It was globally renowned and I had read up on the authors who were going to appear. Elizabeth Gilbert would be there – author of *Eat, Pray, Love*, the book that changed my life and led to me writing my memoir, *Cheat Play Live*. But some of my favourite non-fiction authors from around the world would be there too: Lemn Sissay (*My Name is Why*), Jung Chang (*Wild Swans*) and the author of a book I'd just read about war reporter, Marie Colvin – journalist Lindsey Hilsum (*In Extremis*). I couldn't wait to explore the famed 'pink city' of Rajasthan alongside my literary heroes.

When I started talking about it in Agonda, the Brit Pack at the bar started oohing and aahing at the prospect of me experiencing 'the real India' (which was, I later discovered, code for 'the really poor India'). I was given to understand that it was a much dirtier, poorer, visceral experience than our sanitised-for-the-Westerners Goa. I was to prepare myself for the shock of seeing dead bodies and defecation on the side of the roads.

Hannah and Dave had travelled through Jaipur and Pushkar and had found it challenging, but they said I definitely needed to visit Pushkar, it being their favourite Rajasthani city. I had planned to fly to Jaipur then go by train straight to Udaipur, but I decided to break my journey for two nights in Pushkar. It was on the way, anyway.

On the plane to Mumbai, I prepared myself for the sights I'd been told to expect. *It must be really bad*, I thought, *for everyone to be warning me about it.*

At Jaipur airport, I walked through the marble concourse to be met by a young Muslim man called Sharukh who had come to transport me to the Pearl Palace Heritage *haveli* (townhouse) I was staying at. It was near the legendary Diggi Palace where the literature festival was taking place (for the last time, as it turned out). His tuktuk had bright-blue leather seats with red hearts stitched into them. The frame of the tuktuk was bright red – it was the happiest machine I'd ever seen.

Sharukh told jokes as we hurtled across roundabouts, narrowly missing cows wandering by, as I stuck my head out of the side of the tuktuk and 'wowed' at the terracotta-pink buildings of the city. By the time I alighted with my case at the Pearl Palace, we were firm friends and I had arranged for him to be my driver for my whole three-day stay.

My room was gorgeous: hand-decorated from floor to ceiling in a riot of colour in Madhubani style – black line drawings of gods and goddesses filled with ochres and reds and hot sari pinks. The hotel had been restored in full Mughal style with decorated golden archways along its corridors but with finely wrought carvings of deities on the doors to each room. Mine featured Lord Shiva and his wife, Parvati. I thought of Shubham and wondered what he'd think of this place.

The next morning, after a continental breakfast in the small breakfast lounge outside my room, I met Sharukh outside. He was on his phone, wearing a bright white long kurta over white trousers. He was gleaming like an angel in the Jaipur morning light.

"We go the festival!" he suddenly exclaimed, snapping his clamshell phone shut and jumping into the tuktuk.

I'd opted to wear a Gita outfit – paisley patterned loose silk trousers and sandals, worn with a T-shirt, modesty scarf and a denim jacket. The morning was cool although the day was destined to be hot.

The main drive to the Diggi was along an unremarkable dual carriageway but as we slowed in the traffic near the festival venue, I spotted a 'barber shop' against the palace walls. A man had set up shop there by hanging a small mirror from the wall and setting a blue painted chair in front of it. He was wetting and cutting another man's hair. *Such a simple idea*, I thought. Here, lots of things were outside that would otherwise be inside – people, mainly. It made me think about how much we hid away in my home country, and that necessity (due to the weather) had become a national habit.

Sharukh dropped me off at the gates to the Diggi – an 18-acre sprawl of Mughal buildings and gardens built in the 1860s – and I joined the throng pushing its way into the entrance, which was lined with policemen and women smartly dressed in tan shirts and trousers with berets. The crowd, making its way between a strand of stalls selling everything from jewellery to chai, seemed to be made up of gregarious Indian students and a sprinkle of confused-looking Westerners. I showed my pass and was ushered under an archway into the pink terracotta palace.

The first item on the printed programme for the day was '*Morning Music*' and I stood and listened to a group playing classical raga on stage. The 'auditorium' was tented, rather like the outdoor area of St Anne's Church in Agonda at Christmas, with bright pink patterned fabric billowing over the heads of the listeners.

I quickly found a chai stall and checked the rest of the programme for the day: a session on '*Writing The Lives of Women*' with biographers, Bettany Hughes, Benjamin Moser, Jung Chang, Lindsey Hilsum and Hallie Rubenhold. As I was fresh from the writing of my own life, I was keen to hear what they had to say. Jung Chang was the rock star of autobiography and I couldn't believe she was there: she had written about three generations of Chinese women, ending with herself. *Wild Swans* had been translated into thirty-seven languages and sold over 13 million copies, but it was banned in her homeland, China.

And then, in the afternoon, the author who'd had such an effect on my own life, Elizabeth Gilbert, was in conversation with Howard Jacobson, Avni Doshi, Leila Slimani and Chandrahas Choudhury on the subject of writing fiction. She spoke about grief and the inevitability of encountering suffering in life: "It will come and find you. And then, it will knock at your door." Once again she was able to access and articulate what was in my heart with her words: grief had knocked relentlessly at my door for years.

When I met Sharukh at the end of the day, I was giddy with a feeling I'd never experienced before – the feeling of being at a book festival without working. For once, I'd been a punter – someone who loves books – just listening to her favourite authors talking about their craft. In a Rajasthani palace – bliss. The city itself reminded me a little of Bologna in Italy where I'd spent a week every year of my working life at the Children's International Book Fair. Its cloistered streets were seen here in Jaipur, with even more life and colour within them.

After a morning at the festival the next day, Sharukh took me around the major sites of Jaipur: the Amber fort, the Jantar Mantar observatory, the Sisodiya Rani gardens and the towering honeycombed Hawa Mahal, made from pink and red sandstone. The Mahal stood opposite Sharukh's favourite chai place and we joined the crowd hovering over one man who was stirring blackened spices into milk in a pan, pouring the contents into small clay cups. It made me think of queuing at Starbucks or Costa, but with a much more interesting-to-watch barista and better drinks (and better recycling – the clay cups get used again and again).

"Tomorrow morning, I will take you to the stepwells," Sharukh said, his eyes gleaming as he slurped his chai loudly in the street. It felt like we were standing outside the latest cool, pop-up bar in London, with all the chaos of frantic customers around us. "My friend has a cloth shop there – you will like it."

"Now remember our deal, Sharukh," I said recalling our unexpected stop-off at his 'friend's' jewellery shop the day before on the way back from the festival. "I know you need to take me to certain places on the tourist route but I need you to know that I won't be buying anything. Don't leave me in there – I don't want to waste time in shops when I could be seeing exciting cultural things."

"Ok, ok, I understand..." he replied laughing. "But you might see something you like. Just take a look."

Actually, I'd bought an aquamarine beaded necklace from his friend the day before, so I'd shown that I could be persuaded. Rookie mistake!

The next day, Sharukh drove slowly around the stepwells – something I'd never heard of or witnessed before. They are famous in Jaipur and in other Indian cities – giant openings in the ground with stepped walls where, historically, locals descended to collect stored water. In this desert landscape, these '*baoris*' had been an essential part of life but now they were largely disused.

I loved the way the angle of the sun played with the geometric angles of the stone steps. They made me think of the Jantar Mantar the day before – home of the world's largest sundial and a host of other astronomical instruments made from stone (*jantar mantar* means 'calculating instrument' in Sanskrit). Each *baori* was nestled inside a network of endless stone archways concealing labyrinthine dwellings, with exposed stonework giving away the secrets behind ageing plastered walls. The area was one of the most stunningly beautiful places I'd ever seen, glorious in its distressed state.

I'd begun to notice on this trip that India was a place where things were allowed to age gracefully. There was no constant replacing of old with new and more of an acceptance that tarnish and peeling is just another phase of an object's life. It made me realise what a culture of 'new' I lived in. Everything had to be new all of the time, including people. It was exhausting, trying to keep up with it. Decluttering my flat of all the unwanted 'new' had given me a new lease of life. I'd even recycled myself: newly sober and silver-haired, I felt as though I'd been born again in my fifties.

As we walked through an ochre-coloured courtyard, Sharukh said hello to an old woman in a yellow sari who was coming out of her front door with a plate full of chapatis. Her big brown labrador was sitting outside and as we passed, he lifted a paw at us in what was literally a high five. I managed to get a shot of him doing it before we passed under a curtain of brightly coloured and gold-bordered silks the woman had hanging over a line. Sharukh translated the woman's parting words in Hindi for me: *"The dog waves when he wants his lunch!"*

Finally, we reached the cloth shop that Sharukh had warned me about. I didn't want to buy anything (mainly because I didn't want to add extra weight to my luggage) but I agreed to go in because he was duty-bound to take me there. He waited outside and was already talking to another driver when I was shown into the ground-floor block-printing area by a tall guy called Ravi. Ravi had his long hair pulled back in a ponytail and he was wearing a beautiful suit. As he showed me into his workshop, his team were carefully pressing a carved wooden leaf design drenched in royal-blue dye onto cream linen, all by hand. It was beautiful to watch such craftsmanship in progress.

And then we ascended the stairs to the fabric shop, passing floor after floor of the building. It got darker and darker as we got higher. On each floor I spied young men moving around silently and I was suddenly filled with The Fear. Had Sharukh brought me here for another reason? Why was I following this ponytailed young man into a dark building in an unknown city, filled with other men? A familiar fear spread through my legs and made me feel faint

– I'd felt like this before in solo-travel situations in other countries. Oh god… What was going to happen to me?

Ravi turned round as we reached the top floor of the building and could see that I was visibly distressed. "Is everything ok, madam?" he asked as we walked into a room full of rolled hand-printed fabric.

I thought about being polite for a split second but decided to be honest. "No, everything is not ok. I am very frightened. There are all these men in the building and I don't know where I am."

My rational self knows now that if Ravi had indeed been a villain, this would have been the worst thing to say to him, but I think in my heart I knew he wasn't.

"Oh madam! I will make them go away immediately! We want you to be comfortable."

Leaving me with one of the said young men, who started unrolling fabrics he thought I might like, Ravi disappeared for a few minutes. I made appreciative noises, because the fabrics were beautiful, but there was no way I could carry any back with me, sadly. I couldn't wait to get out of the shop and back to Sharukh and the tuktuk.

Walking back downstairs after about half an hour, having successfully avoided buying anything, I looked behind me as I went. I saw the bodies of young men slowly re-emerging from behind rolls of fabric. It was as though the walls were alive. Sharukh told me that Ravi had told all of his staff to hide while I was in the building to make me feel comfortable.

On the way back to the haveli, Sharukh announced that he was from Pushkar, and he would take me there the next day in his tuktuk and visit his family at the same time. I thought it was a bit strange, knowing that tuktuks can only go at a maximum speed of 40 miles per hour and the distance was nearly 100 miles/150 kilometres but I thought, *Well, he must know what he's doing*. I thought it might be fun.

The next morning, bags packed and ensconced on the red leather seats in the tuktuk, we stopped after only five minutes of trundling through the city at what appeared to be a chai truck stop. The place was filled with upturned oil drums being used as seats, with men driving a range of vehicles from tuktuks to lorries all parked up under a flyover.

In a matter of minutes and one clay cup of chai, Sharukh had negotiated with the driver of a very smart businessman's car for him to drive me the rest of the way. The money I'd paid Sharukh had suddenly migrated to the other man and I was passed over like cargo, with my bag, into the new car. Again, my gut told me I would be ok – the guy was wearing some sort of official driver badge and seemed tame enough. And I was glad not to be on the massive freeway above us in a tiny tuktuk. I waved goodbye to Sharukh and said hello to air-conditioning and reclining seats.

Pushkar was not what I expected at all. I'd been told that it would be an oasis after Jaipur, but when we drove past ragged-looking camels with their owners waiting for tourists on the outskirts, I immediately felt a longing for the tuktuk and Galta Ji. Galta Ji is a Hindu temple complex outside Jaipur that has become synonymous with its colony of monkeys. They posed for the tourists – I got a shot of one looking wistfully over the desert plains of Rajasthan while clutching a piece of hot pink silk – but they were free to roam and lived happily there.

We pressed on to where I was staying – a hotel lodge on the outskirts of the city. I'd need to get a taxi in and out of the city, but my room overlooked fields where I could see women in saris working. Aside from the noise made by wedding

guests who were slowly taking over the venue that night, it
was a peaceful place to stay.

I got a taxi into the city as the sun was at full strength
over Pushkar Lake. There was a small terracotta temple in
the middle of it, with a single tree growing next to it. Groups
of people and *sadhus* (Hindu holy men) walked around the
lakeside *ghats* (broad steps), contemplating a sacred bath in
the holy waters.

I found a chai place with clay cups and sat on an another
upturned oil drum in the shade. It was in the main marketplace which was mainly geared towards tourists but en route
to the most sacred Brahma temple, where I'd removed my
shoes and paid my respects along with everyone else there.

Everywhere I'd walked that day was filled with either
market-stall garishness or ascetic pilgrimage and I couldn't
quite square the two things. How could such rampant
consumerism (and tourist bars) sit alongside so many of these
holy places? And then I thought of the Vatican in Rome –
that does quite a good job of it already.

I found stalls that sold items similar to the ones I'd seen
and bought from Gita, but they didn't look or feel the same. I
bought a mirrored bag knowing she would question me
intensely about how much I'd paid for it and tell me she
could get a better one for me.

I couldn't rid myself of the feeling that Pushkar was like a
Hindu theme park. I'd felt more spirituality in the eigh-
teenth-century streets of Jaipur or the beach road of Agonda
than I had here. Why wasn't I feeling the same way as other
friends who'd visited it?

I walked to the other side of the lake and decided to
watch the famed sunset, which was accompanied by bells,
drums and chanting. Shubham video-called me from Agonda

and told me he missed me and I so wished I could've shared this moment with him, as a friend at least.

"And what?"

"I'll see you when I get back," I said, unable to hold a conversation above the din.

"See you, my crocodile," Shubham answered, never having got the hang of 'see you later, alligator' (although I secretly preferred his version).

I wished he was next to me, holding my hand and felt a pang of longing for Agonda.

As the sun disappeared behind the buildings across the lake, I decided to carry on walking round it and look for a tuktuk back to my hotel. I quickly got lost in the maze of streets as darkness fell and was drawn like a moth to the flames of *puja* just inside a temple, with bells clanging, drums beating and a priest holding candles aloft outside, gesturing across the lake. I later discovered that the sound is intended to create the *Om*, the sound of the universe, of the sun. The cacophony is intended to remove obstacles, Sudhir told me, to clear the mind of distractions. It held me rapt as I walked from one temple to another, witnessing a similar practice going on in every one.

I knew that my old drinking self would have found a bar with Brits in it and I'd have got drunk through fear of the unknown and fear of being by myself. But this new me felt comfortable wandering the streets in the darkness, with the sounds of spirituality to keep her company. Perhaps I liked Pushkar more than I thought.

The next morning, I took a taxi to nearby Ajmer station and waited for the commuter train to Udaipur – the White City, named after its marble buildings. The city was calling to me with its glittering lakes and shining palaces.

I stood on the platform expecting something of the real India to show itself. Trains seemed to be the places where friends had seen the worst things, so again, I prepared myself. Then a beautiful old turquoise train pulled in, slowly, the doors opening to reveal distressed brown-leather reclining seats and a chai man going up and down the aisle.

As I took my seat, a young man popped up to sell power boosters for phones and another sold hot pizzas from a delivery bag. I loved this pop-up economy – it made more sense for a place like India, where the country (or rather, continent) was too big to wrangle into one distinct system.

I'd seen something of it in Agonda when sitting at the bar one day after Shubham returned from the ship. A young man pulled up on a scooter with a huge leather satchel slung across his body. In turn, each member of bar staff went for a *tête à tête* in corner of the bar with him. I'm ashamed to say that my first thought was that he was selling them drugs.

"He works for the bank," Shubham said, putting me straight. "We're paying our wages to him, a little every time."

Of course! The main banks were miles away so it made sense to send someone out on a scooter to hoover up all the cash from everyone. There were loads of scooter businesses already in Agonda, including Flipkart, Amazon and the man from Jio who could sort you out with a SIM card from his satchel. To my suspicious Western brain, they looked like scammers, but they were just doing business the way it's done there: nimbly, in person and in cash.

The train journey was uneventful and I was almost disappointed not to see anyone defecating. Instead I paid £7 to get to Udaipur and travelled in air-conditioned chair class, one of nine seat classes on Indian trains, akin to a standard seat in the UK. I guess if I'd been trying to do it ultra-cheaply, I'd have gone second class (no A/C and wooden benches) or general class (unreserved seating, no A/C, bars across windows), but why would I do either of those? I found the incessant 'I did it cheaper' competitiveness among British tourists annoying and distasteful. To me, it smacked of slum tourism and insulted those Indians that couldn't afford to travel any other way.

I had chosen another haveli in Udaipur – the Little Garden Guest House – with planted courtyards and stained-glass windows echoing the style of the forts I'd visited so far. The owner, Akshay, lived with his family in the house next door and sat talking to me for a long time about the loving restoration they'd done on the 250-year-old Little Garden, each room filled with cushioned love seats and Mughal art, crisp white linen and sunlight shafting in through deeply cut arches in the thick stone walls.

My room was simply best I've ever had in a hotel anywhere around the world. I'd booked a suite because there weren't any single rooms left and I decided to treat myself. As Akshay showed me up the narrow stone steps to my second-floor balcony, I felt like I was lost in Verona. These Rajasthani cities kept reminding me of Italy for some reason.

On one side of the balcony there was a love seat filled with cushions sitting against cool distressed stone, and next to it a separate modern bathroom, a short walk from the main bedroom. Akshay creaked open the bedroom's thick, carved, double wooden doors and there was my bed with its crisp, white cotton sheets. The stained-glass arched windows let diamonds of red, yellow and blue fill the white space with their colour.

Eager to explore the alleged roof garden above my rooms, I followed Akshay's instructions and continued up the stone

steps at the side of the balcony and unlocked the wooden
door at the top. A blast of sunlight temporarily blinded me
before my eyes recovered and found that I was standing on
just one roof among hundreds in the city. Langur monkeys
perched around the edges of each one, surveying me and the
roofs around them, no doubt wondering how quickly they
could get to the one that had food on it. They ignored me
once they realised I had nothing with me, just like dogs.

I could hear the sounds I'd heard in Pushkar here, the
clanging of *puja* bells coming from all around the city. I later
found out that they were coming from the high concentration
of temples in this, the old city, with the largest of all – the
Jagdish temple – only metres away from where I was staying.

I turned to go back down to my room and gasped with
delight. The City Palace was right behind me, towering over
the city – its warm magnolia walls blushing in the late afternoon sun. I couldn't wait to get inside and feast on its
mirrored halls and stained-glass sanctuaries.

Wandering around the city in the early evening, I found
myself on the marble steps of the Jagdish temple, head
thrown back, marvelling at the multi-storey carved
stonework. I left my shoes on a rack at the top of the steps
and padded quietly into the main temple where a shrine to
Lord Vishnu, carved out of black stone, was set deeply inside
the sanctum.

A *puja* was taking place and I stood behind the worshippers, anxious not to appear voyeuristic, although I was taking
everything in with every sense I had: the intense chanting as
worshippers processed to the sanctum, their hands passing
over a bowl of purifying fire; the smell of the burning incense
as lamps filled with fire were swung in front of the deity, the
supreme being of Hinduism, the creator of the universe. I

noted that his eyes bulged and stared out at the congregants, like many of the deities I'd seen in Pushkar temples. On my return to Goa, I asked Sudhir why their eyes were shown like this. "It's an expression of their energy," he said.

Looking for something to eat, I found myself on the other side of the temple in Lal Ghat – like Pushkar, Udaipur had a string of 'ghats' surrounding its five lakes. Lal Ghat sat beside the largest of these, Lake Pichola. The restaurant I found was called Doctor's Café, run by a young entrepreneur called Sheikh who showed me to its roof terrace overlooking the lakes. He was tall and handsome in jeans and a black leather jacket, the owner of this café and a tour business across the road.

As night descended, Pichola's shores were twinkling with light. I decided I would go on a boat trip first thing the next morning, after a delicious Doctor's pizza and a good night's sleep in my cosy room. Sheikh offered to give me a tour of Lake Badi and the surrounding countryside in the afternoon.

I was in bed by 9.30pm but woken at 10.30pm by the clanging of gongs and bells which went on for several hours. Once again, the temples had swung into life at night, just as they had in Pushkar, and I vowed to wander around the following night, taking in the sights and sounds at closer quarters. I remembered Sudhir's words again: "*It is to clear your mind of thoughts and distractions." Well, it certainly does that*, I thought.

The next morning, the breakfast room was filled by me and a bunch of Chinese tourists. Akshay told me they were having a hard time because of the news about something called 'coronavirus' which had allegedly started in a wet market in Wuhan.

I stepped out of the haveli in another pair of Gita's best

loose silk trousers, a matching top and my denim jacket and bought a masala chai at the shop on the corner. It came hot and sweet in a clay cup from a silver-haired man in white kurta and trousers. He was making fresh samosas in a huge shallow wok for the passing morning trade and I sat watching on a by-now familiar upturned oil drum as people stopped to pick theirs up on scooters, on their way to work. *Just like an Italian on a vespa picking up an espresso and a tramezzino to go,* I thought, warming to my theme. Signs for *'rabri'* covered his shop – a North Indian sweet dish made with milk, sugar, cardamom and nuts. I made a mental note to have a lighter breakfast the next day, just so I could try a samosa or rabri.

The waters of Lake Pichola sparkled in the bright morning sunshine but the air was cool. As I arrived at the docking area to one side of the City Palace, I could hear my mother's voice in my head saying 'coolth' – her word for that particular blend of hot sunshine and colder air. I bought my ticket for a lake circuit and a visit to the Jag Mandir (Lake Garden) palace on one of the islands in its middle and boarded the boat with two Indian couples who were clearly on their honeymoons. I decided to style it out and sit at the front, smiling at the boat captain, who described where we were going in an extremely serious, official manner. We pulled past the lakeside edifice of the City Palace, whiter now in the crystalline light. That would be tomorrow's adventure.

There wasn't very much to see at Jag Mandir, other than bustling staff preparing for what seemed like a wedding. It had featured in the 1983 Bond movie, *Octopussy*, along with the Taj Lake Palace, as Octopussy's home. I completed two circuits of the palace, stopping to take pictures in its ornamental gardens and asking a security guard here and there to take a photo of me on one of the marble benches. I was pleased with my Indian silks in the photos when I checked my phone later. I wondered if I could wear them on the motorbike trip I'd planned for the afternoon. I longed to see more of the Udaipur outside the city.

Sheikh met me at his tour shop after lunch and wheeled his Enfield motorbike around to the front. Tying all my scarves, beads and bags securely about my person, we sped off, leaving the old city for the more modern suburbs, which seemed to be full of wedding shops. I liked the way Sheikh rode the bike, mindful of the speed we were doing – I would remind Shubham that we didn't have to go everywhere at warp speed, especially around Goan bends.

We arrived at Lake Badi and Sheikh stopped so I could take photographs at a small white domed platform. He told me that the villain's lair in *Octopussy* had been the Monsoon Palace we'd just passed, perched on top of a hill. But I wasn't interested in Bond history, I wanted to see where Sheikh had grown up.

The sun was setting as we rode along country roads, past farms, cropped fields and through quiet villages. "This is my home," Sheikh announced proudly. Children waved at us from outside their houses and we passed an old man walking on the road carrying a huge bundle of twigs and branches on his head. I remembered what my friends had said about the 'real India' and noted that I'd seen all of these things in the quiet farmland around Agonda. It was an insult to the people who lived in Goa to claim that their lives were somehow inauthentically Indian.

The next day, I saw the produce grown in those fields in the marketplace – a clearing in the tangle of streets leading downtown, away from the quiet backstreets of the Little

Garden. Fortified by a masala chai and two samosas from the corner shop, I decided to see what all the fuss was about – the market, I'd been told, was truly a sight to see.

Just the walk there had me falling in love with the glorious faded grandeur of the city. Every turn down a different street gave me a snatched view through wooden doors into the courtyards beyond: a child playing with a plastic jug, two puppies playfighting, a row of coloured silks hanging on a line. It reminded me of the back alleys and winding streets of Venice where much of the life was hidden behind doors, where lives were lived beside water. It turned out I wasn't the first to say that Udaipur reminded them of Venice.

I found the market in full flow and just like Chaudi, there sat a row of women in saris behind baskets filled with hypersized vegetables and piles of herbs and roots I'd never seen before. The women cried out as I passed, asking for pens (I think). I would bring some back the next time. For there had to be a next time.

A man in a kurta and a bright-orange scarf stood behind a wooden cart with beautifully arranged green beans, studded with bright-red flowers and sitting on red oil cloth. There was such pride in the presentation of the produce – and rightly so, because fruits and vegetables like these were not seen everywhere in the world. I wasn't there to buy, but one day I hoped to be, staying somewhere with my own kitchen. For that moment, I satisfied my retail urge with a pair of royal-blue, peacock-feather-design velvet slippers. Another purchase I'd have to get through the Gita interrogation.

The day after my visit, Akshay told me that people protesting near the marketplace had been beaten with bamboo sticks by the police for protesting against anti-working-class laws. Many of the shops were closed and the temples remained quiet. He warned me against venturing back to that part of the city. "Better to remain in the tourist areas," he said. Even glittering Udaipur had its dark horses.

I spent the next day at the City Palace, roaming its dazzling array of palaces-within-palaces, with their mirrored, tiled and painted halls and coves. I peeked through windows over the lake and the city and stood in front of stained-glass windows, marvelling at the colours like a child bewitched by Christmas lights.

Instead of the usual audio guide I decided to hire a human one, Dattaraj, who knew the zigzagged corridors (built that way to deflect surprise enemy attacks) like the back of his hand. The whole complex – the largest palace in Rajasthan – was 400 years old, he told me, built and added to by Maharana Udai Singh II and his successors.

As I stood in the Sheesh Mahal – the Palace of Mirrors, I thought about a visit I'd made to Versailles in France as a dance student. Now, as then, I felt drawn to the reflected light bouncing around the warren of rooms, but this time it was heightened by the Rajasthani sun.

AGONDA, SOUTH GOA
FEBRUARY–MARCH 2020

FIVE DAYS AFTER MY ARRIVAL BACK IN AGONDA, I HAD not seen Shubham. While I was away in Rajasthan he'd video-called me several times, saying how much he'd missed me and my hopes had built for a rekindling of our romance, but when I was actually there, he was nowhere to be seen. It played into a lurking fear of mine – that I only mattered to him when I was unattainable, that what was driving our passion for each other was distance. If I was too convenient, I was less appealing.

It had happened before with a man I'd met during the final years of my marriage. I'd met David – a Mancunian – at Cannes Film Festival and we'd kept up a sexting relationship for a couple of years afterwards, me in London, him in San Francisco. When I finally turned up in The City on a holiday with work friends, he'd pretended he was in the UK. It was only much later that I found out that he'd been hiding from me. Since then I'd encountered other men who only liked texting me when I was obviously away. Perhaps the unattainability was the driving force behind their desire. I decided to not contact Shubham and waited to see what he'd do. Nothing, it transpired. It was purely a friendship, after all.

I settled back into my routine of early morning walks on the beach and working on my laptop at Simrose during the hot afternoons. I would be continue to be single Lisa – there was no point in expecting any man of any age to do anything, it only led to disappointment. Part of me felt relieved at the enforced alone time but I was heartily sick of being tugged around by the heartstrings. I needed a clean break and I couldn't seem to get one.

The sound of drums from the north side of the village heralded the start of Shigmo festival – Goan's own special celebration of spring and an abundant harvest to come. Marshall told me that the Hindu men of the village would be visiting every Hindu household with drums, songs and fire-crackers, signalling abundance to each house in turn. I read up about the festival and discovered that it was a fusion of Holi, the Hindu festival of colour with which Shigmo ends, and a community carnival. It had its roots in the home-coming of warriors, hence the military rhythm of the drumming.

As I walked up and down the beach in the evenings, I was desperate to see what was happening in the houses that lined the north side of it but I didn't have the courage to nose around. I finally heard from Shubham who was busy with his father and the men of his own community in Palolem. They celebrated Shigmo slightly differently; every village had its own rituals, Shubham told me. I felt annoyed that I couldn't enjoy the festivities with him. Then I wondered, *Why can't I go?!* I was determined to make it happen myself.

I'd met Rocky (aka Vaishal) at Kopi Desa – he was a local at the bar and a Hindu – a tall, well-dressed man in his thirties with a goatee beard, quiet and respectful. One night during the festival, I told him how much I wanted to witness Shigmo and he offered to take me to a family event that evening.

I threw on trousers and a kimono from Gita and wrapped a shawl around my shoulders, determined to be respectful, and waited for Rocky to appear outside the Red House. We sped on his bike to the north end of the village and joined a group of men drumming outside a house that was sitting behind the row of shops. I hadn't really realised that behind the strand of shops on the beach road, there was a host of local houses connected by labyrinth of passageways. From that moment on, my eyes were opened to flashes of bright paint adorning Portuguese-style one-storey villas, and children peeking at me over sleeping dogs in the alleyways in between.

The men wore pleated orange hats, perhaps reminiscent of the homecoming warriors, and some of them – a security guard from Simrose being one of them – were wearing red-tinsel creations with a tail hanging at the back of their heads. The drumming and singing would reach a crescendo before firecrackers were set off in front of the amassed smiling families on the verandahs of their homes. Rocky told me to step back as the drummers needed to file out of the passage to go to the next house, which belonged to members of his family.

After the ritual, I was given food and a place to sit just outside the house, while Rocky and the men of the family ate as a separate group. The women remained inside, peeking out at me, as their pet white kitten curled up by my feet. I felt happy that finally, I had had an insight into some of the cultural traditions of Shubham's life at home, even if I couldn't experience them with him.

However, I felt sure that I would be able to celebrate the festival of Holi with him and prepared myself for coloured-powder-filled gaiety on a day that celebrated the renewal of broken relationships and the blossoming of love.

When I turned up on the morning of Holi for breakfast at Love Bites, Rahul and Sally had already covered themselves in coloured powders. Sally painted my face with them in a tribal way, with striped markings on my cheeks and forehead.

"What's Shubham doing today?" she asked as they prepared for their celebrations.

"I don't know," I replied sadly, feeling sorry for myself that yet another festival was passing by without him.

I went back to my room and took a few selfies of my painted face, to reassure the people in social-media-land that I was still living the dream and then cried. I hadn't heard anything from Shubham and he eventually messaged to say he was in Palolem for Holi. A few hours later he posted a picture of himself with his friends, who were all covered in coloured powder, laughing.

I was done.

I'd befriended a man from nearby Cola, Krishna, who was the owner of a resort that sat beside the river mouth there. I was helping him with some business ideas and he'd offered a stay in one of his huts to me as thanks. I needed to get away from Agonda and its festival disappointments.

Quite apart from the situation with Shubham, I'd started feeling like I couldn't fit in with the British drinking tribe. They had their own routine of late nights, sleeping in and sunbathing in the afternoons that was the opposite of everything I wanted to do – I craved early mornings on the beach before the hot sun came up and and early nights to make those early starts even more possible. As the Brit Pack congregated in the evenings at Kopi Desa to move on to the 'corner bar' which stayed open late, I'd make my excuses and go to bed, happy to leave them to it. I was transitioning out of drinking culture and I was realising what an impact it had on the shape of your entire daily routine, either at home or on holiday.

I packed an overnight bag and took a tuktuk outside the church to Cola. On one of the winding roads en route, we encountered a couple who'd had an accident. They were from Hyderabad and the woman had lost control of the scooter on a corner. It was my worst fear about riding a motorcycle and here was the evidence – it was so easy to get very badly hurt.

My driver ushered the couple to a nearby bench outside a villa on the corner – it was almost as if it had been placed there for that very purpose. They had torn the skin off their knees and arms – they'd actually got off quite lightly, given that they'd slid across the road.

The driver immediately suggested that we took them back to Agonda and I sat with them as they shook with shock – Dr Furtado at Agonda Clinic near the Red House would look after them. She'd looked after me when I was bitten by beach dogs the day before my yoga training. I'd had to have a series of rabies injections just in case. It had been close to monsoon and the dogs got angsty at the encroaching lack of food.

We were quickly on our way again and once at Cola, Krishna showed me to my hut on the other side of the river. It's shallow waters host swimmers and kayakers away from the rough waves. I'd previously felt uncomfortable at Cola, having taken a boat trip there to find restaurants closed to anyone who wasn't staying. It was almost like it had a big '*KEEP OUT*' sign on it and I'd got hot and bothered on the sand with nowhere to shelter until the boat returned to collect me. But here was a hut just for me, shaded by palms with a balcony overlooking the river. Inside it was decorated with simple printed fabrics on the bed and floral plastic sheeting in the bathroom. Cold water only. It had been very hot so I didn't mind. Much.

I planned to read a book and eat alone in Krishna's restaurant, overlooking the mouth of the river. Sunset had now passed and the deep fuchsia afterglow was well in place in the sky above Cola. I wrapped one of Gita's colourful pashminas around my shoulders and settled down, feeling at peace with myself. I enjoyed being on my own – other people, especially men, just complicated everything. Even mosquitoes were a welcome absence – Cola didn't have many because there were no cows around. It would be a night of peace and solitude away from the beeping horns, biting creatures and barking dogs of Agonda.

"And what...?"

It was Shubham. At 9pm. He'd been given the night off from work and had come to find me. I couldn't help but smile but attempted to reset my face into a picture of seriousness.

"Well, this is a surprise..." I said, sarcastically.

"I wanted to see you," Shubham said, placing his rucksack on the table. He was obviously planning on staying over.

"That makes a change. I went to Shigmo last night," I said defiantly, as he pulled up a chair.

I hated the idea of being held back and enjoyed proving that I didn't need to wait for anyone to make things happen in my life.

"Rocky took me. It was really good. His family were really welcoming," I said, forcing my point, attempting to make Shubham a little jealous.

"I wanted to be with you, babe, but I am the only son in my family and I have go to the houses and the temple with my father."

"Did your father throw the coloured powder over you?"

"That was my friends. I saw them at the te—"

"I'm sick of this, Shubham. We agreed to be friends and then you called me in Rajasthan saying how much you missed me, then ignored me when I got back, and now I'm the only woman in Goa not celebrating Holi with her man. Let's just go back to friends. It's not working."

"I'm sorry, babe. I just have so many people calling me – family, friends—"

"I know, I know, you only have time to see me at night. Well, you know how I feel about Nighttime Girlfriend. And now here you are again, at night."

"I got here as early as I could. I was bringing us pizza from Kopi Desa but the box slid off the bike on the way here and I had to go back for it. It was no good – it all came out on the road," he said sadly.

"Well, I've already eaten anyway. I'm going to go to bed early because I'm getting up early for a jungle walk."

"Can I come with you on your walk?"

"You'd be prepared to get up that early? It's 7am," I said, waiting for him to back out. "It'll be daylight..."

"I want to go with you. It'll be ok. I have that type of talent," Shubham said, grinning.

———

I'd arranged to meet one of Krishna's staff at the restaurant at 7am. We would walk upriver to the Shree Laxshminarayan temple at the other end, trekking along the path at the side of the river, sometimes having to step through its shallow waters.

After an awkward greeting – him being an unexpected guest – Shubham chatted happily in Konkani to our guide (a friend of Ram's) while I took in the misty morning among the palms and cashew trees, glad I was wearing sturdy rubber flip-flops. Small rice fields emerged in a clearing up ahead and we tightrope-walked along their edges, ankle deep in a low mist over the water. The sun's rays were starting to push through the trees creating a fresh apple-green glow over the water. For me, sunsets were overrated – this was the time of day when the magic happened.

Finally, we reached the bright white temple with its stained-glass lotus-flower windows. We stepped out of our shoes and went inside. Immediately I became transfixed by the statue of Nandi at the back of the cool white marble space. He stood within a carved wooden casing, a human with a bull's head, his palms pressed together in prayer. Nandi is traditionally the guardian of Kailash, the mountain home of Lord Shiva, the supreme Hindu deity who destroys and then recreates the universe. His mudra, or hand gesture, was *namaste* – an acknowledgement of the divine light that exists within all living things and connects us all. I found it immensely calming to see it, his thumbs pressed to his heart.

In Hinduism, these gods represent aspects of universal laws and characteristics. To worship Ganesha the elephant god, for instance, is to pray for the removal of obstacles. This made so much more sense to me – a set of stories and characters that illustrated and illuminated the world around you, but didn't demand that you believed in their fiction. Having been brought up in the Catholic tradition, I found this system of representation and symbolism much easier to put my faith in.

At the end of our temple trip, we were met by another of Krishna's staff in a jeep and drove the bumpy track back to Cola for breakfast. Shubham and I grinned at each other over masala chai.

"I really enjoyed the walk with you," Shubham said, stirring sugar into my chai.

"I enjoyed having you with me," I replied, "in daylight."

"I will try hard to make time for you in the daytime, my Lisa. I have wanted to call you every day but I think you are busy."

"But I've been waiting for you to call! Every day!" I cried.

"I'm sorry for everything. You are special," he said, reaching for my hand. "You will always be special in my life."

In this peaceful setting I could see Shubham more clearly: a young man who was still learning how to navigate the world. He hadn't yet reached twenty-eight, the age at which I had found full maturity, a sudden awareness of my adulthood and all the responsibilities that came with it. For me, it had felt like a switch flicking – I saw a different face in the mirror. I knew that Shubham still had this moment to come and was perhaps on the road to it right at that moment.

But I still wasn't sure if it would be there with him when it happened.

During March, the news about the coronavirus was reaching a crescendo. I was talking to friends at home about whether or not I should come home early – I wasn't due to fly back until April – but a slight panic was building in the Brit Pack community around me. We'd sit on our laptops at breakfast, nervously surveying flight prices and checking the news at home.

I toyed with the idea of staying in Agonda indefinitely – could I live through monsoon? I was used to rain – I was Welsh after all – but I had a feeling that I would feel miserable on my own. I knew that if a pandemic was declared then I might be cut off from Shubham who lived in another village, and I'd be reliant on Marshall and Saluzhina's hospitality. As lovely as they were, what would happen if 'foreigners' were seen to be the carriers of the virus – a view that seemed to be gaining momentum in the conversations around me? For one thing, I didn't want to put my hosts in the position of being marginalised because of their association with me.

At the same time, my birthday was approaching and I looked forward to the distraction, a break from the roller-coaster of coronavirus drama around me. On the day itself, I decided to walk on the beach as usual, waving at the young man on the mahogany horse who now sped past me each day, trailed by dogs.

I called into Love Bites on my way back, for breakfast and a chat with Rahul and Sally. I played with Ocean the dog when the sound of an Enfield pulling up outside distracted us. Shubham appeared, a white box balanced on one palm, his helmet in the other. He was smiling.

I gulped back tears as I opened the box to reveal a birthday cake with a message to me iced on it. It had slid to one side of the box as Shubham had ridden back from Chaudi with it, but I didn't mind. I loved it, with all its squishedness. I don't know why but I'd had years of making my own birthday fun, with friends and partners all coming along for the ride but all the arrangements left up to me. Cakes had only ever been bought for me at work by my teams, and no one other than them had ever bothered to surprise me with anything. This simple gesture filled me with such joy and the memory of it still does. Shubham's shy smile and the cries of delight from Rahul and Sally as they witnessed the moment. We all sat round as I blew out my candles and made a wish. I wished that my life had been filled with more of this joy.

Shubham's plan for the day was to take me to a place called Assolna. After a half-hour drive on the Enfield, we sat in a restaurant on the banks of the River Sal and ate fish curry. A tiny puppy played at our feet and hoped for fish snacks. The sunlight reflected off the river into our smiling faces. Shubham took pictures of me against the bright blue walls of the restaurant.

There, and on the ride home during golden hour, I felt happier than I had ever felt. We returned via Canaguinim, the location of our dream life together. After sitting and dangling our legs off the wall there, we sped to the red stone outcrops of Cabo de Rama fort in time for sunset. I wanted to tell Shubham I loved him but I didn't want to say something I'd regret, especially if these were to be our last days together.

I decided to protect the sanctity of this golden moment and not say anything at all.

I didn't know if I'd made the right decision to return to the UK just before lockdown. The thought that I had made the wrong one plagued me, not helped by the chorus of voices I was hearing in messages from friends in Agonda who were telling me things were ok there after all.

I found it hard to work out what the truth was – so many people who lived there spun fantasies about their lives, I could never tell. They contradicted themselves in their panic to validate their own choice to stay – one minute I'd get a frantic message about police on the beach wielding sticks, the next a message saying everything was really chilled and people were hanging out at the beach unrestricted, implying I'd made a mistake to leave.

I had left because good friends had implored me to and in my heart, I'd known it was the right thing to do. It was the right thing to be on your home turf during a pandemic, even just in terms of fighting the war against the virus together. The following week saw lockdowns in both the UK and India and Shubham being confined to his home with his family. I knew that if I'd stayed, he wouldn't have been able to see me or look after me. There were roadblocks with checkpoints monitoring traffic between villages and stopping any unnecessary travel so we couldn't have seen each other. I'd have survived the pandemic, but I know those monsoon months would have been extremely difficult for me, not least because of the incessant rain.

I managed to book a flight back to Gatwick that would

get me back in the UK the day before lockdown. I spent my last evening saying goodbye to everyone and every animal I knew on the beach, and I did it with Shubham's hand in mine. I have two photos of that evening, after the sun had gone down: one of Shubham helping Nitesh and his boatmen pull his boat in (he's smiling at me) and the other, a blurry one taken by Shubham, of our footprints side by side in the sand.

At that point, I had decided that this beautiful, shining human was not going to be mine. It was unfair to make him choose between family, friends and me, if that decision was not easy. It should be easy, I reasoned.

I forced myself to mentally photograph every second of that last day because I knew it would very probably be the last time I would see him, and the last time I would be in Agonda. I couldn't bear to go back there if Shubham were to get married to another woman. I could be happy for him without putting myself through the torture of witnessing it.

Before our last beach walk, I'd cried my heart out in his arms. *He doesn't know I'm not coming back*, I kept saying to myself. As I said goodbye to Sweetpea, Sanjo and Zimbo my throat closed up in an effort to stop a torrent of tears from falling. *They don't know I'm going either*, I thought, but maybe they did. Dogs sensed things.

At 3am the following morning, I felt Shubham's velvety skin under my hands for the last time and jumped into a taxi. I can still see his expression as he turned to his bike for the ride home.

Goodbye, my love.

THIS CHARMING MAN
ENGLAND

WORTHING, WEST SUSSEX
MARCH–APRIL 2022

THE FRESH COLD SPRING AIR OF WORTHING SEAFRONT helped me get some distance and perspective on everything that had happened in India over the past few months. I'd reached peak happiness around my birthday, and once again, it felt like part of my soul was being ripped out when I left Shubham and Agonda. But at the same time, I wondered if the universe was trying to tell me something. I told myself that the pandemic was a sign that Shubham and I weren't meant to be together forever.

I'd already begun to formulate a theory that humans relied on 'foreverness' in relationships way too much anyway – I had a sneaking suspicion that we weren't wired that way, that society was forcing us to follow a rule that didn't fit our genetic make-up. I tried to think of that helpful Dr Seuss saying, *'Don't cry because it's over, smile because it happened.'*

After all, how many fiftysomething women got to experience the things I had experienced? How many women of my generation had been lucky enough to know and feel the love and desire of a Shubham? How many of them had experienced life and work in India? I tried to feel grateful, in a yogi way, for everything that had *already* happened, not the things that were not going to happen in the future.

At home, well-meaning friends made faces that said, "Well, it was never meant to be, was it?" or maybe that was what I chose to read in their expressions. I'd told some of them about the issues I'd had the previous seasons, with Shubham's disappearances and mood swings, and they said they hoped for better for me. I'd hoped for better for me too, but I'd found it on my birthday and in Cola and Assolna. A different Shubham seemed to be emerging in those last weeks and days of my time in India but now I wasn't there to witness the full transformation.

I was staying in rooms with a family in Worthing, just as I had done in Agonda. I wanted to recreate my life there almost exactly – a house near the sea (check), a friendly family (check), animals (dog and cat – check) and affordable rent (check). My belongings stayed in storage and I existed as I had done in India, with just a few cold-weather items I'd left with a friend in London. I got them couriered down – they were left on the doorstep in case of infection.

I kept my routine of walking by the sea each morning, knowing we were allowed out for exercise once each day. As time went on, I increased it to twice a day – I wasn't going near anyone, so what harm was it doing? Nerys the lurcher refused to come with me, a stranger, but I reasoned that people with dogs would have to go out twice a day, so I took my imaginary one for a walk.

I also did what I had to do for my own mental health – I turned off all the messaging from Agonda (apart from my Indian friends) and unfriended where I needed to on social media. I knew that a few of the friendships had come to a natural end and decided to cut all ties. The voices requiring validation that staying behind was the right decision were getting too loud for me to bear.

I couldn't believe that the family I was staying with allowed me into their home straight away, given that I'd come through four airports to get there. As she showed me into my beautiful big room in her Edwardian home, decorated in cool greys with white-painted restored furniture, my landlady Elsa reasoned that they were more likely to be the ones infecting me: they'd been in London only a week before with someone who'd tested positive. As it was, none of us caught the virus during the whole of lockdown.

We existed as a tight-knit family group – Elsa, husband Dave and son Finn, Nerys the dog, Bob the cat and me. I paid extra for them to buy food and cook for me and I led online evening yoga classes in their living room while Elsa joined in on her mat and Nerys groaned on the sofa. I decided that Nerys was my Karma Yogi, even though her assistance was entirely based on her intermittent 'breathwork'.

Elsa and I worked at our laptops on the thick oak kitchen table in the huge kitchen Dave had renovated while Dave homeschooled Finn in the lounge. Elsa was a designer and understood what I was saying about problems with my editorial work – I was still finding it hard to manage my emotional responses to certain clients who seemed to trigger something in me over the smallest issue. Often, my second walk of the day was a stomp around the pier to release my anger. She reassured me that I just had very high standards and got frustrated when other people didn't match them.

Yes, I thought. *That's it. I just have very high standards.*

I'd been an avid hiker before the pandemic and part of my reasoning for coming to Worthing was its proximity to the South Downs. In addition to my daily walks by the sea, as the lockdown rules began to lift, I started some forays further afield onto the South Downs Way with my friend, Paula. We'd take flasks of tea and bags of chocolates to share on the way. We must have walked the same circuit a thousand times – Worthing to Cissbury Ring, Lancing Ring, Shoreham by Sea, then back along the seafront to Worthing. I revelled in the greenery and cool air that I'd been longing for in the hot, dry, red dust of India.

Not long after the lockdown restrictions had been lifted on 4 July, the first 'Freedom Day', I'd just finished teaching a yoga class online when a message suddenly appeared on my phone from Luke, a 50-year-old guy I'd met on previous group hikes. We'd chatted and got on well, but I was wary of him. He was good-looking and charming and I'd jokingly named him 'Hiking's Most Eligible Bachelor' when I mentioned him to my friends. I'd noticed that he was charming to everyone – he had that ability to talk to everyone in a group in a way that made them think he was extremely interested in them individually. I imagined that some gullible women might fall for that and make a fool of themselves.

Luke's text asked me if I'd be happy to have a call with him, as he had an exciting offer for me. I texted Paula, *"Wtf? What can he want?"* She was as surprised as me, but I was also a little flattered that he'd thought of me. I texted back an agreement to a video call later that day.

Luke told me he was researching some long-distance paths in the UK for the adventure company he worked for.

He was also an Instagram influencer, using his six-figure following to showcase his photographs. He told me that his main audience was older women like me – somehow I wasn't surprised.

He was hiking the 62-mile Northumberland Coast Path over four days, staying at B&Bs and guest houses en route between Cresswell and Berwick Upon Tweed. Luke wondered if I'd like to join him.

I couldn't believe it. *Why me?* I wondered. But after the lockdown I craved adventure and hiking somewhere far from the south coast and said I'd love to join him. *Why not?* I thought.

I concluded that Luke must have chosen me as his hiking companion because I would provide insights as a member of his core demographic and the adventure company he worked for, which catered to older solo travellers. *It must be that*, I thought, especially as he'd clearly done his research on me, mentioning various things I'd written about on my blog and details from my author bio. Yes, this request had come about because I'd be useful to him, I concluded, and I'd get something out of it too: a wonderful coastal hike. I'd been to parts of the Northumbrian coast as a university student as a few of my friends were from the North East. I knew it had charm and charisma: a bit like Luke.

After the call, Paula and I spoke and she asked me what the sleeping arrangements would be. I hadn't even thought to ask. I'd assumed it would be separate rooms and felt a bit awkward having to ask the question. He confirmed: '*Of course! We'll have our own rooms.*'

I decided to tell Shubham what I was doing on one of our regular video calls. I told him that this was a friend I'd met through hiking and that it was just a friendship trip, nothing more, because it was. He seemed to take the news well and I read it as relief. It had crossed my mind that while the universe was forcing Shubham and me apart, it might also be offering me a more age-appropriate contender in his place. This would, in turn, release Shubham from any ties to me. He would be free to explore a relationship with a nice Indian girl his own age.

My friends were excited for my trip. Although they didn't say it in so many words, their response to it implied that they saw it as an opportunity for me to move on from my 'holiday romance'. Even I had started to think of it in the same way. What was I even thinking, trying to have a relationship with a man half my age who lived halfway around the world in a completely different culture? Here was someone who was more age-appropriate and into the same things as me. I would see how the trip went – perhaps Luke really did only want me along as a hiking guinea pig, but part of me began to hope that he wanted more.

NORTHUMBERLAND COAST PATH
AUGUST 2020

I met Luke at Kings Cross and we chatted like old friends all the way to Morpeth, where we'd be spending the first night of our trip. We both had neatly packed thirty-litre rucksacks with us; we were leaving for the trip at the start of August – so I didn't need much in terms of bulky items, despite having to carry our things from stage to stage of the walk.

I learned that Luke was half-Dutch on his father's side – and I realised was responsible for his surf-guy good looks: blue eyes, golden skin and thick dark-blond hair.

I knew the trip would be good when he suggested going for a late-afternoon walk near the first B&B – I'd spent so much time with men who never suggested doing anything. I'd always been the director of every relationship I'd ever been in, with them relying on me to initiate all the fun. Finally, I was being taken somewhere by someone.

We had adjoining rooms in the one-storey B&B, a small corridor and bathroom linking the master bedroom and a smaller room. I immediately insisted that he should take the master room and pushed aside any disappointment when he immediately accepted my offer as though the issue had never been in doubt. *Fair enough*, I thought, *it's his work gig.*

Luke name-dropped the company he was working for wherever we went on the trip and it opened the doors to great service and rooms. I revelled in it and decided that at long last, this was the sort of treatment I deserved. Luke was shaping up to be an ideal candidate for my perfect potential relationship.

In a local pub that evening, I asked Luke why he'd asked me to accompany him. Quick as a flash, he replied: "Your intelligence. I knew I would need someone to walk with who would be able to hold a conversation."

That got my attention. A man who wanted me for my brain. It was a new sensation.

The next morning, on the first stretch of the coast path from Cresswell to Alnmouth, Luke took pictures of me in my red waterproof jacket in the sand dunes. There was a fine drizzle accompanying our start, but it didn't dampen our spirits. I hiked ahead, feeling strong and compact with my red rucksack on my back. Luke had been surprised by my packing light – I suspect he'd been expecting me to bring heels and a load of beauty products. That was the old Lisa.

Before the trip, Luke had mentioned a surprise he had in store for me. It was special accommodation for our second night. *A man has organised a surprise for me!* I was delighted. As we hiked and chatted along the broad sandy beaches and up and down the grassy dunes, my romantic fantasy began to build, especially when I turned round to see Luke's eyes roving over my body in my Lululemon yoga leggings and tight-fitting top. It was a look I'd seen in another lover, just after my separation from my husband. I was flattered by the desire flashing in a man's eyes, but at the same time it felt like a look of conquest, of ownership. I packed the niggling doubt away and decided to run with the romantic fantasy instead.

We arrived at our destination – Alnmouth – and met Dale in the café he ran with his wife. Their small collection of three designer 'camping cabins' right on the edge of the beach was my special surprise. We took showers in a cubicle in the café as the huts didn't have any and flung our bags into the back of Dale's golf buggy for the ride up to them.

Dale was a bear of a man – black hair and beard with distressed T-shirt and jeans – and while he drove us up to our hut, he told us how the pandemic had affected his business, which had only opened in May the previous year. He'd been fully booked when lockdown hit, his huts being used in the winter months by artists and writers on retreat, but he then faced multiple cancellations. Now the world seemed to be opening up again, and his grin belied a sense of great relief at the prospect. He showed us around our hut, which was situated on a hill overlooking Alnmouth beach.

"Only one bed!" I exclaimed, as a look passed between the two men.

Inside the hut was a tight little space, beautifully decorated in Scandinavian style, with blankets and logs for the wood-burning stove and a tiny toilet and kitchen area. The one double bed was wedged into a space at the back of the hut and only a slim sofa offered another space to sleep. Dale showed us where the local deli had placed our complimentary parcel of food and departed for the evening, leaving us to sort out our sleeping arrangements.

I waited for Luke to suggest he took the sofa but no such offer came. I thought about taking it myself, but the bed looked so cosy and inviting.

I texted Paula and told her about my predicament. She was unsurprised.

"*It'll be fine,*" I said. "*I'll just stay on my side of the bed. It'll be like 'It Happened One Night' with Clarke Gable and Claudette Colbert.*"

She wasn't so sure.

Luckily, I'd packed a shapeless huge T-shirt to sleep in. I didn't want Luke to think that I was trying to entice him in any way.

After a supper of bread and cheese from our complimentary hamper (we both avoided the wine) we took to bed. We stayed up chatting for hours, making each other laugh, and I found myself not wanting to go to sleep at all. We had to get some sleep, as Luke's alarm was set for sunrise – the perfect time for a photoshoot – so we decided to settle down.

His arm 'accidentally' touched mine as we moved around, trying to get comfortable for the night. And then we kissed.

It wasn't as good as I'd thought it might be. For one thing, he tasted very strange and I didn't like it. My ex-husband and subsequent lovers had tasted good – I always thought that it was a test of good gene-matching – if you liked the taste and smell of someone, there was a good chance you were biologically matched to become parents. I decided to overlook it – it felt good to be desired by someone almost my own age.

But then he started to speak in a low, slightly threatening voice about what he thought I would like – to be dominated by someone like him, a real man, he said, after all those boys I'd had. I lay there wondering how the laughing, joking Luke I knew in the daytime had turned into Christian Grey at night. I decided to go along with it, as he seemed to be enjoying it – people were allowed to have a dark, fantasy side to them; as long as it didn't translate to real-life aggression, what was the harm?

"I need to admit something to you," he said before we went to sleep. "I don't just like you for your brain, I like your arse too."

We woke at 5am the next morning and Luke went straight outside with his camera. I put the kettle on to boil for tea and took two mugs and blankets with me to join Luke at his vantage point over the sea. It was one of the most romantic moments of my life, handing over a hot mug of tea to a smiling man, all traces of Christian Grey gone, a lens to his eyes and the click of his camera punctuating the cry of curlews from the sands below.

I pulled a patterned blanket around me and smiled into the rising sun. Yes, this is how a relationship is meant to be: a creative man of my own age by my side, appreciating me not only for my body but my mind too, and sharing a sunrise, with no hangover to spoil it. He was like Clint Eastwood in *The Bridges of Madison County* – but I hoped this blossoming affair would last for more than four days.

Over the course of the next stretch of the hike, a very hot Alnmouth to Seahouses, I told Luke that I'd been worried about his intentions, my concerns that he was a charmer who applied the same approach to every woman he met. I had a nagging feeling that he just wanted a hiking fuckbuddy and I was the nearest easy target. We both laughed those ideas off, because they seemed so absurd in the face of what was happening, which was an undeniable, real connection in an undeniably real romantic setting.

That day was so hot and unfeasibly long (we were trying to condense the route and fit in a boat trip at the other end) that I ended up with blisters all over my feet. Luke suggested I should be properly fitted with new boots when I got back – I'd been getting blisters every time I did more than one day of hiking and it was so disappointing to be held back at the very moment I'd just got going. I agreed to his suggestion and made a mental note to act on it when I got back to Worthing.

The next day, Luke had a scheduled interview at Bamburgh Castle but I decided my feet needed to rest. The castle was within walking distance of Seahouses – most of it along a beach – and the rest of that day's section, which would take us within sight of Lindisfarne (Holy Island) wasn't the most exciting stretch, so I would take a taxi to our next accommodation. To help my feet, I decided to walk to Bamburgh Castle barefooted on the sand, and then return the same way after seeing Luke for tea and cake at the castle café. I could complete it all in flip-flops.

In the end, Luke decided to sack off the rest of that stretch himself and catch a bus to Beal where I was waiting in our pub accommodation. We had dinner and planned our next stretch, Lindisfarne to Berwick, our final destination.

After Alnmouth, we'd reverted to twin-bed rooms and I'd decided to hold off doing anything more than kissing until I was more sure about him. I'd jumped in too quickly before – usually as a result of drinking – but this was the first time I was encountering a potential partner sober. I was going in with a clear head.

"I need you to know that I have had someone special in my life, In Goa," I told Luke the next morning on Holy Island. "He's called Shubham. He's much younger than me but it was more than a holiday fling. We meant something to each other. He'll always have a place in my heart."

Luke nodded silently as we walked over the island and didn't ask any questions. He'd already told me about his ex-girlfriend, whom he'd moved in with but then promptly broke up with. I didn't ask questions either. I'd just needed him to know that I was still processing a previous relationship, if his intentions to me were romantic. I figured that no guy wants to hear anything about a love rival so I shut any further conversation down.

We were visiting a coffee roastery on Lindisfarne. We instantly regretted not staying on the Island overnight, having been warned off it by someone advising on our trip. After too much Colombian caffeine, we clambered over the tidal island, eager to see as much as possible before the incoming tide prevented our departure.

Hobbling into Berwick at the end of the final day (I was determined to complete the trip on foot, with lashings of Vaseline coating my burst blisters, on Luke's advice) I felt excited about the future. Luke and I had forged an incredible connection over the past few days and I hadn't immediately given myself to him and made the situation awkward. I'd been honest about Shubham and Luke hadn't run away.

Yes, he'd shown himself to have this Christian Grey alter-ego, but I put it down to a personal fetish. It was a dark horse I hadn't encountered before, and I was tempted to laugh at the vocalisation of it, but I realised it was something he was into. Perhaps I could overlook it. Everyone had them.

I had that swirl of excitement and desire in the pit of my

belly as we boarded the train back to London the next day –
the kind of feeling you get when a new relationship is beckoning. When we parted again at Kings Cross, I readied
myself for the 'let's get together again soon' conversation, but
it didn't come. Instead, I witnessed a transformation. The
man who had looked at me like I was the only thing he
desired in the whole world, suddenly smiled as someone
would at a new acquaintance they had just met over a coffee,
and promptly waved a very PG-13 goodbye. It was as though
we had just been on a day hike together with one of our
groups.

I took the steps down to the Underground wondering
what had just happened but decided not to judge anything
based on one incident. Maybe he was just tired and keen to
get back home.

I travelled back to the south coast in a state of near-bliss,
trying to get the sight of Luke's neutral smile out of my mind
and replace it with one of his grins from the coast path. Still,
a little voice inside me was wondering if I'd simply been a
convenient hiking companion, a lockdown love interest. The
company he worked for dealt with international travel and
were it not for the pandemic, he'd have been abroad. Was he
making the most of his enforced stay in the UK by adding a
woman into it?

We began to chat by WhatsApp again over the following
weeks. It was strangely restricted to certain times and days
when he was free – he said he had family and work commitments. I tried not to wonder why he didn't want to get in
touch with me more readily – I had work commitments but it
was easy enough to text someone in between them. I didn't
want to be checking my phone for a text from any man at
my age.

Meanwhile, Shubham began a campaign of sending me regular '*Good morning*' and '*Good night*' messages and video-calling me from time to time. He'd left overly joyful comments on the pictures I posted of myself and Luke, and although I sensed that he was overdoing it, I assumed he was fine with what was happening and this was his way of endorsing it. I told myself that he was relieved that I was finally off his hands.

On one video call, I told Shubham that I'd started 'seeing' Luke and he told me he just wanted me to be happy. He said it over and over again, as though he really meant it. I was blown away by his mature response and assumed that he might be relieved that I'd set him free. Perhaps there was a girl in Goa. Perhaps the universe was right after all.

"If he is better than me, then you should go with him. I just want you to be happy."

"But he isn't better than you, Shubham. He's just different. I am allowed to have him. We are not allowed to be together but he can offer me a future."

"I just want you to be happy."

"I just want you to be happy too."

"Goodnight, my crocodile."

"Goodnight, Shubham."

CUMBRIA WAY
LAKE DISTRICT, OCTOBER 2020

In the autumn, Luke began messaging me about another plan – this time the 70-mile Cumbria Way. He would be walking it in October, and he asked me if I'd like to join him again since we'd got on so well in Northumberland. I was delighted to accept and we began messaging excitedly about the plan. The government had reintroduced the 'rule of six' coronavirus measures in September, but it would only impact our plan minimally.

The relationship had moved on since our first trip. I'd already booked myself a solo hiking break to the Isle of Wight a few weeks after Northumberland and invited Luke to join me. He didn't seem excited at first – he'd already been to the Island – but eventually he decided to join me. I had walked the Freshwater Way several times alone – unlike Luke, I was someone who valued going back to the places I loved over and over again, rather than constantly searching for something new. I wanted to show him 'my' island. I also wanted to take the relationship to the next level and decided it would happen that weekend.

My body decided to intervene to try and stop me. After months of no period, I had a strong feeling that it was about to stage a big return. In the summer of 2019, I'd been told by the doctor that my periods would likely stop in the next few months because my blood test showed a low level of oestrogen. I had a vague idea that I was in the stage before menopause: perimenopause. I'd been warned by other menopausal friends to expect a 'Biblical flood' from time to time before my periods stopped completely and I was nervous about it happening that weekend because I'd had the telltale cramps for a couple of days. Well, let's just say that our 'reunion' kicked things off big style. The only thing missing was Moses.

We were due to go for dinner on the first evening and I had to rush back to our Air BnB twice to change what I was wearing. It was like being a teenager at school again, worrying in case my 'leak' could be seen. I even had to tie a sweater around my waist. In the restaurant, Luke chose a table with leatherette seats so I wouldn't leave a stain. It was horrific. He took it all in good stead and we joked about this being a good 'period drama'. It turned out that the drama was confined to that first night – things cleared up quickly after that.

He must really like me, I thought, *if he's willing to overlook this hideous occurrence and make jokes about it.*

The weekend was fun, but I had a nagging feeling that 'my island' wasn't good enough for Luke – it wasn't exciting enough. It made me question why I was always going back to pastures old when everyone I knew was always after the new place to visit. I decided to try and break my old habits. I wouldn't go back to places like Agonda again – or Dahab or Bodrum, which I'd visited multiple times. I would find new places, perhaps with Luke by my side, instead of flying solo.

———

Towards the end of October, we arrived in Carlisle for the first leg of our Cumbria Way trip and were put up in a sensational suite in the best hotel in town. We ran around like excited teens on Spring Break, bouncing on the sofas and beds and spinning around in the huge kitchen. The apartment was bigger than my flat in Worthing – the one I'd moved into to avoid having to bring Luke into my lodgings with Elsa and Dave. (I'd felt like their teenager bringing a boy home for the first time.)

We were walking the route in reverse – normally people started in Ulverston and ended in Carlisle but Luke had decided after doing some research that the reverse way was better.

Day one went well – we were still in 'frolicking' mode, enjoying the slow disappearing act of the city, the path making its way into the countryside around Carlisle and slowly heading up, up and up towards the Lake District. The weather was mild but cloudy and it seemed like we would repeat the joy of the Northumberland trip, with only heavier packs to mark the difference, containing fleeces and waterproofs for the inevitable weather changes.

Day two was wet. Very wet. We only made it out of the tiny village of Caldbeck to the Lingy Bothy near High Pike, before we had to shelter there out of the torrential rain. It was fun inside the stone hut while we watched the wuthering weather do its thing outside, but less fun once we started walking again. Luke was following our route on an app. Someone else whom we called 'the man' had already walked the Cumbria Way and we were following in his virtual footsteps. But what we didn't realise was that sometimes 'the man' got it wrong.

Once the rain had abated, but not completely stopped, we donned all our wet-weather gear and started the tricky descent into the Glenderaterra Valley. Luke started picking his way down ahead of me, and I struggled to get my footing on the slippery stones and deep mud. It wasn't until much later after the trip that Luke admitted that we'd strayed off the path at that point.

He'd been in a strange mood all night and all morning because the place we'd stayed in Caldbeck was bad. After the luxury and glamour of the Carlisle hotel, we'd been given a terrible room with missing lightbulbs and no toilet paper – possibly the worst room I've ever stayed in.

After a set-to with the owner, Luke had discovered that in an act of desperation after the pandemic downturn, the owner had offered his best room to another guest. He said that he hadn't been sure we'd turn up – nothing had been confirmed by Luke's company. To top it all off, he promised us a 'superb' meal as recompense but it was basic, to say the least.

It was the only time that Luke and I went to bed and straight to sleep. He was really annoyed – I just felt sad that the landlord had initially lied to us about the situation, claiming there'd been a mix-up, and then finally told us the story of how he'd taken on this new business venture just before the coronavirus hit. It was clear that he and his wife were struggling to keep it afloat.

The further we walked into the valley, the further behind I fell, and the less Luke appeared to care. He often ran ahead on hikes or lingered behind to get the right shot on his camera, but on the previous trip he'd involved me much more in the photo-taking, grooming me as a potential assistant. (It was another reason why I thought he'd picked me to go with him – he needed a caddy.)

But on this trip, something felt different. He was walking way ahead for long periods of time, and not necessarily taking photographs. He wasn't checking to see where I was or how I was getting on and when, on occasion, I did catch up, he muttered something about needing to keep up the pace. Unfortunately, this had the opposite effect on me. I slowed down to a pace I was comfortable with, annoyed with him for this weird race we suddenly appeared to be in. I slowed to see just how far he would take it and at various points I lost sight of him ahead on the path.

I sang songs to myself as I walked, trying to laugh off the situation, and toying with the idea of getting a train home from Keswick. I daydreamed about Shubham, about clinging to him on the back of the Enfield, and how he would never have left me on my own in a situation like this. In my head, I was on my way to the Red Crab restaurant near Cabo de Rama, on my way for a biryani with a man who cared about me.

As we approached Skiddaw House, a landmark up on the slopes of Skiddaw itself, Luke finally decided to wait for me and held out his hand to pull me up a particularly muddy bit. "Well done!" he cried, smiling weakly.

Inside, I nearly exploded with fury. *Well done?! Well done??!!* I was the one who had hiked in Kyrgyzstan, Georgia and Armenia and could take on just as much as he could, if not more. I did not need a 'well done' from a man who was determined not to walk with me. He was positioning my lagging behind as a failure of my fitness, to make himself feel better. In reality, I was lagging because I didn't want to catch up with a man who was treating me so badly.

On the descent into Keswick at Latrigg, we finally fell into step beside each other. The views out of the valley were spectacular in their autumn colour, the bronze bracken just emerging and water flowing in miniature waterfalls to our left. A stream of fell-runners pushed their way up past us, sinews straining with every step. I was fascinated with them, how anyone could push themselves so hard that they'd be prepared to run up and down mountains.

I turned to Luke with an eyebrow raised. "Nice to see you!"

He looked at me, puzzled.

"Well, I haven't seen you for a while," I added.

"Oh, sorry, I just needed to get a few photos. Plus, I've been worried about getting to Keswick before dark."

I wondered why he hadn't simply stated that, instead of trying to 'pace' me like an animal or child. I didn't respond to people racing ahead of me – if anything, it always made me go slower, willing them to knock themselves out with the strain of getting ahead for no reason at all, like dogs choking themselves trying to get ahead of the pack.

But in the end, I decided to shelve my plan of going home. We had a rest day in Keswick planned for the following day and I wanted to enjoy it. The guest house owners, Paul and Nicky, welcomed us to their best room with views over the fells. Order was temporarily restored.

On our rest day we wandered around Derwentwater, the three-mile-long lake that Keswick sits alongside. We took a boat trip, and although the grey skies stopped Luke from being able to take any great pictures of the surrounding fells

(Cat Bells being the most well-known and visible) I loved the slow chug of the boat around the lake, Luke putting his camera down to put his arms around me from behind.

I'm not alone anymore, I thought. *I'm in the world with someone to make sense of me. I fit in.*

But that night, Luke asked me if I was thinking about someone else when we were in bed together. It took a beat for me to answer and he banged the bed with his hand in frustration. I decided not to answer, because I couldn't in all truth say no.

The next morning we met with a friend of mine, an adventurer who had pulled himself out of a life of depression and alcoholism and now ran up fells and cooked on top of them. Harrison would walk with us as far as Langdale and cook a meal for us on the way. Like Dale in Alnmouth, Harrison was a bear of a man – perhaps more of a Norse God – and his grin made for a friendly start to the next part of our Cumbrian adventure. It was a welcome relief to have someone else walking with us – Harrison and I had sobriety in common so we chatted away about our personal stories while Luke scampered around taking pictures.

As we walked, something struck me. There was something so humble and authentic about Harrison, even though he too had a sizeable Instagram following. He didn't flash around in branded adventure gear or name-drop who he'd been working with. I found myself feeling slightly embarrassed in front of Harrison that Luke was the man I was with.

Once Harrison bid us goodbye to catch a bus back to Keswick, Luke and I continued on to our next stop at

Stonethwaite, to a cosy inn for the night. There, it was clear that we both needed some space from each other – Luke quickly showered and left me in the room to complete my ablutions to go downstairs to the bar. I took my time, relishing the solitude and the cosy tweed-blanketed room.

The next day I was left in no doubt that there was something afoot. Once again, while walking through the spectacular Great Langdale Valley and up Stake Pass, Luke walked far ahead and showed no signs of wanting to walk with me. Once again, I employed my walk-even-slower-and-sing-to-myself strategy, trying to enjoy the journey whilst simultaneously giving myself space to work out what was going on.

It started getting dark as we descended into the Mickleden Valley towards our next stop at Elterwater where we were staying at a hostel. We were wet through as the rain had set in and wearing our head torches. I decided I would tackle Luke when we stopped for dinner. I had to nip this behaviour in the bud.

"I've got something to talk to you about," I began, as we were seated at a table in a warm, dry pub in the village, taking care not to spray our raindrop-covered waterproofs on the surrounding customers.

Luke looked surprised.

"I was thinking, that if you'd prefer to walk the rest of this alone, I can help you with it by going home. I'd happily get a taxi to the nearest station."

"What? Why would you do that?" Luke replied, clearly shocked.

A woman at a nearby table was listening in. I didn't care.

"You have walked ahead of me consistently for two days now. You've used the excuse that you are taking photos, but I don't think it's that. You don't want to walk with me. As I say, I can just go home..."

"I'm sorry. I've been really worried about getting to our destinations before dark. It's why I've been trying to go faster, to get us there quicker."

"Well why not just tell me that? Why just run ahead and leave me behind? I've been planning to leave you from just before Keswick."

"I've just been slightly panicking. I'm sorry."

I suddenly saw Luke for what he really was. Not the experienced adventurer, but a man who was used to being led on hikes by someone else, who now suddenly found himself in charge (or so he thought) of me. He was using a navigation app for the first time and trying to appear as though he knew what he was doing.

I reminded Luke that I was used to adventure hiking and absolutely fine with encroaching darkness. I had the right gear, I had a head torch and I liked the moonlight. He nodded and smiled back weakly.

From that point on, all I could see was someone faking it. Not only was his adventurer persona fake, but he was faking his interest in me, and his *bonhomie* was something he could switch off as soon as he reached the point of parting. I'd never seen anyone's face so clearly change whenever we parted to go to our respective homes. He'd go from interested party to passing stranger in nanoseconds.

One day after the trip, while I was working at home, Luke sent me a link to an Instagram post he'd made a year or so ago, featuring the image of a hut he'd stayed in with someone he referred to as his ex 'Mrs'.

I felt sick. It was almost exactly the same as the Alnmouth hut we'd stayed in but it was in the New Forest.

'*You've done this before?!*' I texted back immediately, wondering if this was his MO with all women.

Ha ha, yeah,' he responded, seemingly unaware of any weirdness on his part.

All I could think was, *I'm not the first.*

After Cumbria, we arranged for Luke to come to Worthing to stay with me in my new flat. I wanted him to meet Paula and go hiking with us and a few others on the South Downs.

It was all great – he cooked for us on his first night and as he bustled about in my tiny kitchen, I felt happy and convinced that what was happening was right. *Men don't cook for you unless they're truly interested*, I reasoned.

After a Saturday of hiking on the South Downs we spent our Sunday strolling by the sea. There was something on my mind that I wanted to bring up with him, something about the words he'd used to describe me on the previous day's hike. I'd overheard him referring to me as his *'hiking buddy'* .

On the way back to my flat, I decided to just ask Luke straight. "When you speak to your friends, what do you describe me as?"

"Oh... I'm actually glad you asked that. I—I just want to take this slow..."

I couldn't believe it. The man who'd taken things from a

cold, standing start to sharing a tiny hut on a six-day holiday was telling me *he* wanted to take things slow.

"Are... Are you disappointed?" he asked tentatively.

"No, I mean, yeah... Of course I am."

I couldn't hide it. But I did manage to hide the anger inside me. I'd fallen for it – the oldest trick in the book. A charming man.

It had happened before. I'd had a rebound affair with a charmer called Dean after my marriage ended. Dean and Luke shared some characteristics, including looking at me in a particularly lascivious 'owning' way when I wasn't looking. I'd caught them both doing it. Something in my gut had registered that look on that coast path in Northumberland and bells had been clanging ever since. In my race to move on from someone and be accepted in the world as a woman with a more appropriate partner, I had once again given myself to a man who didn't deserve me. My anger was mainly directed at myself. Clearly my advancing age wasn't giving me more worldly wisdom.

We sat quietly watching TV that night. I didn't know what to say and Luke looked sheepish. I went through the motions of enjoying the last of the weekend, but I couldn't wait for him to leave. Once again, I said goodbye to a stranger at the station.

———

The second national lockdown kicked in in the UK from 5 November so our Cumbrian trip and Luke's Worthing visit had just snuck in under the proverbial wire. We were on an enforced break, and I was actually relieved. It would give me the time and space to consider what I was doing.

I was still in touch with Shubham and I looked forward in increasing measure to his daily 'good morning' and 'good night' messages on WhatsApp. His authenticity suddenly shone like a rescue beacon in the dark.

Luke was largely silent, but when we finally did speak by video call he let something slip. He'd told me he was considering coming to see me again and was talking to his flatmates about the viability of him being in a 'bubble' with me, which would allow him to travel over to Worthing. He told me the argument he was thinking of presenting to his friends: that he had 'needs' that needed to be met. He laughed and quickly brushed over his statement, positioning it as a joke, quickly replacing it with a hasty, "Because I need to see you, of course!" but I knew in that split second that he'd told me the truth. He needed me for sex, as his lockdown love interest, as I'd suspected.

He'd also let slip on a previous visit that his ex-girlfriend, she of the previous hut, had accused him of 'ruining her life'. He told me he'd moved in with her, even when he knew the relationship wasn't going very well. I suspect, like me, that she'd thought the relationship was going well and had the potential to be long-term. Until she realised he had no intention of making it so.

I'd long been fostering a theory that Luke gave women false hope. When I first met him I could see that several of the women in the hiking group thought his attention meant more than it did. One of our group had definitely fallen for it and made a fool of herself trying to make it happen, even though he was in a relationship with the girl whose life he 'ruined'. He joked that this woman had become a bit of a stalker, and we'd both laughed about it. That was, until I realised he'd given her the false hope he'd given me. Unconsciously or consciously, it was his MO.

My anger was growing. I wanted to end it with Luke before the end of the year, but friends convinced me that it would be a bad idea as it would spoil my Christmas. I wasn't sure if it wouldn't completely improve it, but I agreed to hold off until the new year.

On the morning of January 12, 2021, I asked for a call with Luke and we arranged a time later in the day. That lunchtime, he was hosting a Q&A on his Instagram feed and I tuned in as I walked by the sea, as it had been my idea for him to host one. A follower asked Luke what his advice was for experiencing heartbreak and rejection. Given that his entire feed was nothing about his personal life, I thought it was an odd choice of question to include. I wondered if it was a deliberate attempt to make a statement ahead of our phone call. I can't recollect Luke's answer – something about just needing time to get over it – because I was furious that he was bringing the subject up publicly, on that day of all days.

When it came to the call, I'd written everything I wanted to say down and I blasted him with it all, from the irony of him wanting to take things slowly while asking me to go on holiday with him as a first date, to the weirdness of his changing personality at every train station we'd ever parted at. He stared at the screen as I ranted, taking care to add that I didn't enjoy his Christian Grey act in the bedroom either – I preferred real passion. I wished him and his family well and we ended the call civilly with a smile and a wave. I have never felt such complete closure and relief in my life.

I immediately texted Shubham to say it was over with Luke. He called straight back, confused by my texts, thinking that I was telling him I was in an official relationship with Luke. I put him straight. I told him I hadn't stopped thinking about him and I loved him. He told me he loved me too.

"I replay our last days together over and over in my head," he said. "I wish we could ride to Canaguinim, Cabo de Rama and the Red Crab over and over again, 'til our last breath. This time, I will never let you go, my Lisa."

We agreed to be in an official relationship, as far as we could when we were thousands of miles apart and still unable to go public in his community.

Over the ensuing days, Shubham revealed that he had been crushed by my apparent abandonment of him. He had spent nights lying awake and early mornings walking on the beach in the dark. He'd cried while helping his mum in the kitchen, which he'd done to try and take his mind off the situation, but didn't tell her what was wrong. He'd confided in his friends about me and they'd told him to let me go, if I was happy with this new man. But I hadn't been. I'd been trying to be, in order to leave Shubham behind, but he was firmly sitting in my heart, as he'd been from the first moment I met him in December 2017.

I had let society and the responses of friends affect my choices, leading me down a path with a man who'd just wanted me as a hiking fuckbuddy all along. Worse still, my gut had been telling me that was what he was doing right from the start and I'd deliberately ignored it. But in society's eyes, I'd finally found the 'right' person, because he was almost the same age as me, based in the UK and into hiking.

We were a good match, they said, and I agreed. And it had felt almost too good to be true, because it was. Luke had said the right words to reel me in, telling me he liked me for my intelligence, when really, he liked me for my arse and as a vessel for his 'needs'. I cringed at what I had allowed myself to do in the name of a socially condoned relationship. I had not only allowed him to violate me, I had willingly violated myself.

I knew Shubham and I would seem like the quickest rebound relationship ever, but I didn't care – it wasn't a rebound because it had never ended: Shubham had been in my heart all along. I wasn't going to allow my worry over what other people would think direct my life anymore. I knew where my heart lay and it was with Shubham in India. It didn't seem to matter that we were 4,500 miles apart or if he was on a ship – the thread of our connection was as strong as ever.

"I am angry with myself for acting crazy when you were here before," Shubham said, rubbing his hands over his face in a video call. "If I had not let you be Nighttime Girlfriend, you would never have wanted to be with this man. I wish I could do it all over again."

"We will do it all over again," I promised him. And I knew we would.

Very quickly, it was as though Luke had never happened. I unfollowed, unfriended and muted him on all the various platforms we'd been connected on and Shubham and I resumed our daily ritual of morning and evening video calls. Working alone at home that winter, his calls flooded my little flat with Goan sunshine and love.

On 16 January, the UK entered its third national lockdown. I hunkered down like everyone else and largely kept myself to myself, working as an editor on books other people had written during the first two lockdowns. The book I had written in India two years previously lay nestled in a folder on my desktop, hiding its dark horses from the world.

When I was offered the chance to write and edit some books for children myself, I jumped at the chance, but once again, I found myself responding to my client badly, no matter how much I tried to manage it. After every call, I felt a resurgence of the red mist I'd felt in India. Every interaction we had resulted in either intense anger or tears on my side, and sometimes both, and they seemed to be beyond my control. *It's only flippin' children's books!* I'd tell myself, after a post-call stomp round Worthing pier. But somehow they'd turned themselves into monsters under my bed.

I knew I had a habit of 'clustering' my anxieties into one big ball. Early in my career, I'd worked at the publishers of *A Huge Bag of Worries,* a picture book by Virginia Ironside, and the title popped back into my head now, to describe this snowballing effect. I noted all the various issues I was worried about down on my phone: I was worried about burning bridges with clients after outbursts like this; about how I would afford my new rented flat in Worthing on a free-lance wage; about how I'd let myself by duped by Luke (he hadn't quite been blocked from my brain); about how much pain I still had in my shoulder and whether a self-employed life in the UK was what I truly wanted. Was it really the Holy Grail or should I go back to the corporate world?

My ego was being tempted by status and salary again: the jobs market had started to open up and calls were coming through. It would be so easy to accept a role as a publisher in a company again and slot right back into that persona I'd adopted for twenty-five years of my life. But that woman was not the real me – she strutted around trade fairs trying to feel important, drank too much prosecco to numb the stress of toxic office life, and wore glamorous clothes and dyed her hair red, trying to feel young and desirable. I knew in my heart that I was so much happier working at my kitchen table in my leggings with my silver hair tied into bunches and drinking Nosecco, but the lure of that life, with its sparkling towers, still had power over me.

All of these things rolled like relentless waves through my nighttime brain, leaving me exhausted each morning. I'd drag myself out for my usual morning seaside walk, running through all of my topics several times, then have to take myself on an evening walk on the pier to revisit them again after work. As soon as I'd finished picking over the details of one topic until it was down to the bone, I'd start on the next one. I'd find some solace on the yoga mat after work and walks were done but it was getting harder and harder to get myself onto it.

Just as I had in Agonda, I began to take note of the cycle of the moon and its effect not only on the tides but on me. On my morning walks, I noticed that the full moon often meant that the waves were mightier when they crashed against Worthing's pebble beach, so it wasn't a stretch to conclude that my own emotional peaks were tied to it too. After all, humans are around sixty per cent water.

The first person I'd see every morning was Dave in his Cloud 9 Coffee van, which was a converted horsebox on the prom at the end of Heene Road, my entrance point onto the beach. It was painted sky blue with scudding clouds all over it, often disappearing into the horizon completely if you approached it at the right low angle from the road. Dave was always ready with a pun along with my coconut cappuccino and we'd make each other laugh, trying to outdo each other's puns before I began my walk westwards.

Cloud 9 acted as a sort of clinic during the pandemic. We'd all dutifully queue to get our few minutes of chat with Dave, and I would personally get annoyed if anyone tried to involve themselves in my allotted chat time. We all wanted a piece of Dave in his little blue horsebox, a smile and a joke before going back to our everyday lives. Sometimes our chats would veer into the spiritual and the profound – no topic was off the menu with Dave. He was our beach guru during the dark days of lockdown, with his twinkling brown eyes and *Peaky Blinders* flat cap.

One day, I mentioned my thoughts about the full moon and its effects on my mood to Dave. I thought he might laugh at my woo-woo theory, but instead, he showed me a picture on his ipad of the phases of the moon. He too had noticed the waxing and the waning, and the effect on himself and his clients. From then on, I'd tell him how I was feeling each morning and we'd joke about the phase of moon we were in. He was clearly on his own emotional rollercoaster – sometimes disappearing for days and returning with a 'you don't wanna know' expression on his face. But while we all told Dave about our own dark horses, Dave didn't ever divulge his. The daily information transaction was only one way.

One day, introduced me to one of his other customers, Danny, who was also interested in all things spiritual, having also lived in India for a while. He had been a carer during the worst of the Covid care-home crisis in the UK, with over 18,500 residents confirmed to have died in the UK between March and June 2020. Danny had personally witnessed tens of people dying in the home he'd worked in in Worthing over just a few weeks – and that was just one of the many care homes in the town. He now spent his mornings in one of the seafront shelters, gazing at the horizon with a cup of Dave's coffee warming his hands. Our unspoken rule was that we wouldn't talk for too long – we both wanted to have our morning communion with whatever it was out there, alone.

Worthing was a hotbed of woo woo, if you looked closely enough. I already knew about the yoga scene that had been thriving before the pandemic and there was something about the energy by the sea there that reminded me of Agonda. Perhaps it was the light and the friendly people; I wasn't sure, but it was familiar. Except there were no cows paddling in the sea or beach dogs digging for crabs (dogs were banned from certain parts of the beach at certain times of year).

I met my friend Elsa, my now-ex-landlady, at Cloud 9 one morning and told her about my 'huge bag of worries' and my theory about the phases of the moon.

"Interesting... Have you considered hormone replacement therapy?" she suggested, being slightly more pragmatic about my emotional issues than me. "My friend swears by it. Apparently, she felt better on day one. I have a friend who is a receptionist in a surgery where they have an HRT nurse. Why don't you give them a call?"

I said I'd give it some thought. I was still having periods but by now they were erratic, heralded by the Biblical flood in the Isle of Wight. I'd accepted that my body was changing in my early fifties but it didn't seem to be having too hard a time of it. I wasn't sure I was in full menopause and if I was, I was not sure I wanted to admit it.

When I got home, I put the HRT nurse on my *'lifemin'* list on my computer – things I knew I should do but rarely got round to. In my head, HRT came with a cancer risk – it was something only certain women took and I wasn't sure who those women were. My mum hadn't taken it – not to my knowledge, anyway.

I googled the symptoms of menopause and gasped as I realised that could tick off at least six of them: joint pain, insomnia (I'd blamed it on booze but I was sober now and still sleepless), anxiety, mood swings, low concentration (I'd found it harder and harder to start my work and was having to work til late each day to keep up) and thinning hair (I no longer had my shiny thick mane even though I'd stopped using hair dye). The only thing I hadn't experienced was hot flushes and I wasn't sure about sex drive – I seemed to be able to cope really well with having a long-distance relationship so perhaps that was my answer.

But what seriously blew my mind was finding out that oestrogen was an anti-inflammatory hormone and therefore a painkiller. When levels of oestrogen dropped during menopause, women experienced more pain, especially in inflamed joints. *My shoulder!* I'd blamed it all on stress and difficult yoga poses – and there is no doubt they both contributed – but during all that time I could've taken something for the inflammation and pain – HRT.

My mind immediately flew back to the conversation I'd had with the doctor pre-Goa. She'd told me my periods were about to stop because of low oestrogen, but had no point had she said that this might be linked to the joint pain I'd reported to her or that I might want to try HRT. She'd simply given me some eye drops saying I might start to experience dryness (which I did). But my symptoms had never been linked to hormones until now.

I spoke to the HRT nurse, Karen, at the local surgery and

told her that I didn't realise that all my symptoms were related to one thing – menopause. That I'd got so used to living with them that I thought they were a normal part of ageing and it was something women just had to put up with.

Karen told me she'd start me off on two different patches, mimicking a normal cycle and including a period, as I hadn't completely finished having periods naturally. One patch contained a plant-based oestrogen only, the other oestrogen and progesterone. I'd have hugged her if I could – as it was, the pandemic meant that I could only speak to her by phone and collect my patches at a distance, behind a mask. I'd had to conduct my own blood-pressure test before starting. I was to change my patch twice a week on the same days – Sundays and Thursdays for me – and place them below my waist. They would not come off in the shower. If they did, you simply replaced them.

Just as Elsa had suggested, the effect of wearing an HRT patch was almost instantaneous. A feeling of deep calm washed over me, the pain in my shoulder reduced, which meant I could sleep more soundly because the pain wasn't waking me up. The red mists abated and I felt ashamed that I had let them rip through my body for so long. The huge bag of worries seemed laughable, when I looked back at the list on my phone. I had lost all perspective and I began to realise that my symptoms had all been coming on over a number of years, not weeks or months. How long had I been victim of 'age-related crankiness'? How long had I been a stroppy cow and not realised it?

I remembered my mother's irrational mood swings in her early fifties when I was a teenager. I could think of a hundred women I'd met who'd groaned about the same issues as me, completely unaware that they could do something about them. I couldn't believe I'd lived with the symptoms for so long, not being one to rush to a doctor every time I felt a twinge. I'd had X-rays on my shoulder and they just told me I had bursitis (inflammation). Not one medical expert had suggested that my symptoms stemmed from low oestrogen levels and that these could be reduced with HRT patches.

I spoke to Shubham by video call, giddy with excitement, but aware that I was about to tell my 26-year-old boyfriend about my menopausal triumph. But as predicted, he was delighted for me:

"I just want you to be happy, babe. My smiling Lisann."

It was his new name for me – a contraction of Lisa Ann, which he'd seen on my passport. I liked it because my mother once told me she'd wanted to call me 'Lizanne'.

"I just feel like myself again! No more stroppy cow!" I cried.

Shubham looked puzzled.

"How I used to be before ... all angry with everyone. A stroppy cow. Never mind! It's a British thing."

"Ok Britisher babe. I'm happy for you," he said, laughing.

I sent him the cow emoji in a Whatsapp message straight after the call.

In April, Shubham had told me he'd been called up by the agency who handled his cruise-ship work. I couldn't believe that people were prepared to go on holiday in such a tightly packed environment during a pandemic but it seemed that they were. And those people were Britishers – they would be cruising around their own country, served by Goans like Shubham.

My new friends T and Tony (both called Tony and differentiated by the initial) were already planning their return to their favourite ships.

"We love a cruise," T said, the taller of the two men, outside our regular haunt, Sea Lane Café. I'd met them both during lockdown as we queued at a distance for Sea Lane teas and coffees. T was someone who talked to everyone, while Tony stood quietly nearby. T was wearing a palm-tree print shirt and matching shorts. "We've never been to Scotland or Ireland so we'd definitely consider a UK cruise."

Talking to a few new friends at the café, I was surprised at the number of people who went abroad at least once a year but had never explored their own country. Now we were all being forced to take 'staycations' in the British Isles and discovering our homeland anew. I had always embarked on trips in the UK – as a child I'd holidayed in Wales, plus I'd been married to a Scot and explored his homeland and Ireland with him. Being part of a hiking group had opened up even more regions of the UK for me. I knew that once people discovered what jewels lay on their doorstep, they would realise what they'd been missing out on.

T and Tony got particularly excited when Shubham confirmed that his home port would be Southampton. I couldn't believe that he was actually coming to the UK in May, and not only that, just a train ride away down the coast from me. T and Tony knew every inch of the port and town and started recommending places I could take him for lunch during his breaks. I wasn't sure he'd be allowed off the ship.

I was meant to meet Shubham at Heathrow airport, or at least see him there before he would be whisked away on a minibus bound for the ship. But the day before he was due to arrive, a storm hit the south-east of England and the trains were affected.

"I'm not coming," I said sadly, when he finally managed to get wifi at Doha airport midway through his journey.

A friend of his had said that he wouldn't get any time in the airport anyway, so I didn't think I'd be missing out, but it transpired that he had at least half an hour free before the bus turned up. The next day, he sent me a picture of Costa Coffee in Heathrow, where he was waiting for the agency to pick him up. I kicked myself for not trying harder to get there.

But then, an hour or so later, I received a panicked text. Shubham had tested positive at the airport for coronavirus and was being taken to a hotel nearby. He'd been the only one of his cruise-ship cohort to test positive, having tested negative in Goa before taking the flight.

I tried to put myself in his shoes – in a whole new country in the middle of a pandemic, testing positive for a life-threatening disease, and being taken to a hotel where he would be held in isolation for two weeks. I felt helpless but at least he had good wifi at the hotel so we could talk by video call. He'd told his family that he was simply being quarantined as a precaution. He didn't want to worry them by saying he'd tested positive. In any case, he only had a slight temperature. He had none of the other classic Covid symptoms such as a dry cough.

I arranged to come to the hotel with a care package as soon as I could, hoping to at least wave to him through a window. My taxi pulled up at a Novotel outside Heathrow in the rain. The place was surrounded by security staff in hivis jackets and walkie-talkies. It was like something out of a 1980s science-fiction drama. I couldn't even get close.

I handed my care package for Shubham to a security guard who agree to help. It contained a variety of things that I found in a local gift shop: chocolate, playing cards, a big silver S to decorate his room, a pair of socks that said 'PERFECT BOYFRIEND' down the side and some 'Happy Banana' sugary treats to make him smile.

The guard came back to me. "There is no one of that name staying here."

I called Shubham, and through a process of deduction, we concluded that I was standing outside the wrong Novotel. His hotel was on the other side of the airport. I requested the bag be brought back out – for a moment I thought they would view it as 'contaminated', but they handed it back to me and I called another cab.

I pulled up outside the right hotel at exactly the moment when the heavens opened. I pushed open my umbrella and looked up above the portico of the building along the row of darkened windows. Brilliant, even if he could see me, I couldn't see him. My eyes caught a slight movement behind one of the windows, directly above the portico to the right of the building. Something shifted and the window opened a few inches. Three brown fingers extended round the glass and wriggled in the air. My Shubham!

I shifted my position so I could see into the crack of the window to the right. Something was moving. Something white flashed past. It was a smile I knew only too well. My Shubham. We laughed and waved at each other manically for a minute or two, unable to believe that we were only metres apart, instead of thousands of miles.

I pulled myself away to go inside and deliver my care package. Minutes later, Shubham had spread everything out on his bed and sent me a photo of it all. We video-called for twenty minutes, me inside the lobby of the sanitised hotel, Shubham in his room.

I was impressed with the cruise company's choice. I'd been very worried about how he might be treated in these sorts of circumstances, but as it turned out, he was in a new business hotel with all mod cons and all his meals delivered. As his first days stretched into his first week, he started to get into a routine of writing, drawing and yoga. He made friends with the Indian staff in the hotel and they managed get him some local Indian food from Southall. He said they were delivering too many big meals, and he'd had to leave some of them uneaten.

My dark horse turned out to be a secret diary-keeper. He'd brought a notebook from home and wrote in it daily. He told me he'd always done it, and now it formed part of his quarantine routine. He sent me photographs of sketches he'd made of some of my Instagram pictures, including one of the Beachy Head lighthouse on the South Downs Way. I was surprised by his creative talent but I'd also been surprised when he told me he loved to tend his garden at home. Every chat revealed something new about him.

Shubham's dark horses were actually filled with light. The things he kept a secret from the world were the things he now turned to in isolation: nurturing, creating and visualising the world on paper. I was so impressed with his resilience and ability to just get through the days. I knew that other friends had taken a real hit to their mental health during a travel-enforced quarantining, but Shubham just applied the Indian philosophical principles I'd learned in yoga training: when circumstances are beyond your control, the one thing you can control is your response to them. He kept calm and smiled often, simply living through the days, enjoying as much of them as he could, doing everything in moderation. I sent him a bar of Tony's Chocolonely and he ate one piece of it every day. I was so proud of him.

Finally, he was taken by minibus to the port and was able to board his ship where he would be given a guest cabin for another term of isolation. He'd already done sixteen days and how had to do ten more on ship. Yet again, a calm resilience kicked in. When he was finally 'let out', he would move to tiny crew quarters which were at the water line of the ship, next to the noisy engines. How he coped with it all I'll never know, but he did.

In June, I got the urge to see a medium – to see if they could reach the parents I'd lost long ago, my dad when I was ten, my mother when I was thirty-two. I don't know why I felt the need to do it, but the need was strong. I looked up '*Worthing medium*' on the internet and found Miriam. Her brown eyes beamed out from her website, sparkling and energetic. I booked in for an appointment.

Miriam lived on Worthing seafront in a Mediterranean-blue-painted Edwardian house that also housed her partner's chiropractic clinic. As soon as I entered the house she started chattering ten to the dozen. "I'm talking too much! It's like a waterfall once I start. I think you would like the group I run, it's full of people like us," she said in a German accent, handing me a glass of water.

People like us? Who was that? And how did she know I was one of them?

I followed her up the stairs to a spacious living room that

she saged liberally before we began. It smelt wonderful. "Just cleansing the energy of the space!"

She offered to record the session too. I agreed that that would be a good idea. I wouldn't be able to remember everything she said if she carried on speaking at the rate she was going at.

"I can see a young man, possibly your son. He's dark … and very crunchy! Ooh yes – very crunchy indeed."

'Crunchy' was Miriam's word for handsome. I didn't tell her that 'my son' was actually my lover. I wanted to hear what she said about him first.

"He's connected to you but not actually with you. He's close by but you are not able to see him. He's just out of reach. He's an old soul, like you – you have a very strong connection."

In spiritual terms, an Old Soul is not only someone who is wise and mature beyond their years, but someone has lived through several reincarnations. There was no doubt that Shubham was mature. We seemed to understand each other on a very deep level that transcended our twenty-seven-year age gap. We were two sparks of energy that existed in the same universe, and that was enough for us. It didn't matter that we were walking around in markedly different human forms.

I told Miriam I was trying to connect with my parents. After falling silent for a few moments with her eyes closed, she began to describe them to me as they were around the time I was born. Nothing about that moment made me feel sad – I smiled as she told me my mum was knitting (something she did a lot). She gave me a message from my parents to my brother, using words only they would use to describe his childhood. I passed it on to him later, slightly wishing I'd waited until he wasn't driving to deliver it.

And then it came. The moment that changed everything. "They're showing me a book!" she cried.

I knew it immediately. I knew that the book they were showing her was mine.

I had vowed never to publish it, because it contained all my dark horses, all the bitterness and anger I'd been holding on to. I had begun to think of it as a form of therapy for me – a way of processing what had happened in my life as a result of childhood grief. How I'd found myself in an unhappy marriage and eventually cheated on my husband in a misguided bid for freedom. How I'd relied on alcohol to numb my pain and stress from grief and a high-flying publishing career and it had led to bad decisions and wrong turns. Writing the story down had helped me gain some distance on it all and release some of my horses into the wild. But some of them were still stamping their hooves and demanding that I revisit them.

I told Miriam that the admissions I'd made about myself in the book made me afraid to publish it, that there would be a backlash against me because of what I'd done.

"Write from the heart and not your ego," she said. "Go through it and take out any blame or judgement and take responsibility for your actions. Be honest with yourself and your story will shine. It will speak to people who may need to hear its message and no one will judge you because you have been honest with yourself. We are all human and flawed, Lisa. If you're wondering why you're here on this earth, it's to help other people."

At that very moment, Shubham was circling the UK on his ship, taking passengers from Southampton to Dover,

Newcastle, Edinburgh, Orkney, the Shetlands, Glasgow, Belfast, Liverpool and Holyhead. He was seeing more of the UK than most of its residents. Miriam told me that the purpose of this continuous 'orbiting' around me was because I had to complete the book and needed time alone to do it. He would stay away as long as it needed to be done.

Do what needs to be done. The words of my guru in India, Sudhir, that changed my life so simply and completely.

I walked back along the seafront in the late afternoon in a mild state of shock. It wasn't even a question I had to ask myself. I would go back to my book and make it publishable. I would publicly admit that I had cheated on my ex-husband and set my dark horses free so that others might avoid making the same mistakes as I had. I had never been so sure of anything in my life.

DARK HORSES RIDE
WALES • ENGLAND • INDIA

I HAD DECIDED TO WALK PART OF THE WALES COAST
Path when I was with Luke, and even offered it to him as a
potential research topic for his adventure company. But
when we split up, I told him firmly that I was taking this trip
with me, that I wanted custody of my own country. I was
determined to complete that hike before he got to own it in
any way.

The Llŷn Peninsula part of the coast path, running
roughly between the town of Caernarfon in the north to
Porthmadog in the south, was where I had spent childhood
holidays both before and after my father had died, swell as
the nearby island of Anglesey. My memories were filled with
their shallow waters rippling dancing light over vast sandy
bays.

Initially, I had planned to complete the walk alone, but
Paula and I had spent a week the previous September
walking her home path – the South West Coast Path – from
Clovelly to Padstow so we wanted to book another trip
together. We were a great hiking team with a similar vision

for how it would work best – carrying our own things from
B&B to B&B, booking dinners in nice restaurants along the
way. In my head, I wanted to be one of those women who
lived truly in the wild with everything they needed on their
backs, but in reality, I liked my creature comforts every
evening and a nice breakfast to start the day.

On our first day on the South West Coast Path, we
encountered a group of weathered women in their seventies
who were bivvying each night with only a tarpaulin to cover
them and KitKats to stave off their hunger when they
couldn't get a meal in Clovelly. (During the pandemic, many
places were shut or open to bookings only – walk-ins were
temporarily suspended. Plus Paula had pre-warned me that
everywhere shut early in this part of the world.) We were
both in awe, but also glad not to be in their position. KitKats
weren't going to cut it for us.

My Llŷn trip was to be a kind of pilgrimage. I'd long had
a difficult relationship with my home region of North Wales
because I'd experienced the trauma of losing both my parents
there and my grief overshadowed any kind of natural beauty
it had. All my memories were of deep sadness and the grim
grip of 1980s unemployment in a town, Holywell, brought to
its knees.

I'd done everything I could not to visit my hometown
because I couldn't cope with it – I had needed to distance
myself from it while I pursued my glamorous career in
publishing in London. I was not that girl who'd wandered
around alone on the hilltops wondering where her Heathcliff
was anymore. I had made something of my life in the
sparkling south. I was even living in a golden flat in Kensal
Rise and nothing on earth would tempt me back to the
pebble-dashed bungalows of North Wales. Until now.

I'd already begun the rewrite of *Cheat Play Live* and I hadn't expected to enter a huge period of introspection because of it. I hadn't told anyone what I was doing except Miriam, Shubham and the cover designer and I wanted it to stay that way. I didn't want anything or anyone to derail my progress on the book and I knew I was too sensitive to others' comments. If I kept this to myself, I could stay focused, I thought.

I realised the Llŷn pilgrimage was now something I probably needed to do alone but I'd committed to doing it months before with Paula, someone I loved hiking with. I was concerned about how I'd manage my need to be with myself – I'd be communing with my parents and thinking about my book as I walked – but I told myself it'd be fine.

At the start, Caernarfon was a nice surprise, having only the vague memory of visiting its castle as a child. The coast path was studded with a string of Norman-era castles, my 'local' one being Flint Castle. They'd withstood the wild Welsh weather over centuries (and by the care and maintenance from organisations like Cadw – the Welsh National Trust).

On our first evening, getting a surprise early walk-in spot at our intended Italian restaurant, I was delighted to hear the staff all speaking Welsh. I could only speak a smattering of my own language, having been taught it at school and opting to stop at fourteen. It was a matter of regret for me that not only could I not speak Welsh, but I sounded supremely English, having adopted the received-pronunciation tones of public-school England in my publishing career. I hadn't done it consciously – my accent had just slowly mutated until it fitted in with the prevailing one in the offices I worked in. Only a trained ear could detect that I still had a northern hard 'A' in words like glass and bath. I was never going to ask for a 'glarss' of wine – it just didn't sound right to me.

The restaurant stood by the sea, near the castle itself. What I remembered as a grim, grey landscape now sparkled with the light off the water, the grey stonework of the town glowing in the setting sunshine. The town was smaller than I remembered, with more winding streets and cobbled stones. The rooms we'd booked were at the top of a hostel, a renovated stone building where seagulls stood outside the windows. For once, it felt good to be home.

"It's almost like being in a foreign country," said Paula, laughing, still grieving the loss of her international travel plans during the pandemic. "After all, the sun is shining and they're speaking another language!"

The next day, we had our breakfast in the sunshine of a courtyard café near the castle. We decided to start the walk in Trefor, a fishing village a few miles down the coast, as I'd read that the path out of Caernarfon was pretty much roadside until that point. We'd catch a bus instead.

We bounced off the bus and immediately began the steep climb out of the town in the direction of Nefyn, looking back over a long strand of sand backed by stone houses and mountains. The sun was still shining. I almost didn't recognise my own country. As a pair of hikers, we thrived on moving quickly from milestone to milestone, but I realised later that we'd missed the town's harbour and pier and the ancient Church of St Beuno at Clynnog Fawr, a major Llŷn landmark. I made a mental note to go back one day.

We stocked up on supplies in the small town of Nefyn before exploring its beach and part of the spectacular coastline at Porthdinllaen. As we walked out along its Carreg Dhu headland, we noticed that the path thus far had been studded with benches placed strategically among the seagrass, places of rest and contemplation. For us, they provided places in which to eat the cakes we bought at our various stops. "Wales loves a good bench," we said repeatedly, encountering one after another.

We made the decision to stop and restart the hike again the next day back on the headland – we were tired and needed to hike back to the hamlet of Edern to our accommodation. The coast path was still in its infancy so Paula had to fashion a few unorthodox routes to get us off the path to our accommodation and back on it again, sometimes staying in the same place twice because there was nothing at the end of the next day's hike. We'd then have to get a bus, taxi or a lift back to the coast to restart the path the following morning. I realised later that we'd only looked down over Porthdinllaen fishing village and its famous Ty Coch (Red House!) Inn. Again, I made a mental note to go back.

The next morning, further out on the headland in another day of sunshine, we found ourselves circumnavigating what must be one of the most spectacular golf courses in the world. Nefyn Golf Club is a 27-hole golf course taking up pretty much the whole headland, with a view out over the sea to Anglesey and even Ireland on a clear day. It made me feel sad that such a wild and windswept place was filled with men hitting little white balls across manicured lawns while wearing pressed slacks. Why did they feel the need to tame and commandeer the best and wildest places?

Confined to a tiny path at the edge of the fairway, we couldn't wait to get to the end of the course and continue our journey towards our next stop, Aberdaron. Because of the lack of accommodation opportunities, we decided to leave the coast path at Porth Colmon and walk the shorter route inland to Aberdaron. The following morning we'd find our way back to Colmon and continue round again to Aberdaron. We knew from the South West Coast Path that it was dangerous to walk too many coastal miles in one day. Every wrinkle in the coastline added anything up to an hour of walking to the planned mileage per hour.

The section of the coast path forming the westernmost part of the peninsula is called Uwchmynydd (high mountain), marked by its highest part, Mynydd Mawr (big mountain – the ancient Welsh language likes to keep things simple). I was not prepared for this sweeping promontory with its green fields, wild rocky headlands and a large island just in view, to feel so spiritual. It poured over me like a thick mist, enveloping me in its embrace.

Paula walked on ahead as I folded into the feeling, a connection with a place I'd never been to before. I didn't want the walk to end, but we had a dinner booking at 7pm at the hotel we were staying in. I stopped to talk to some horses who were whinnying into the wind near Mynydd Mawr, tossing their heads at my approach. They were all the colours of a chocolate box: dark, milky chestnut and cream. I wished they could run free and take me with them all the way to the top of the mountain.

Sittting behind a rock to get out of the wind, we snacked on fruit and biscuits to boost our blood sugar before the final stretch of the hike and spotted some people waiting on the rocks below. It looked as though they might be staying on the island which was now fully in view. I felt envious, looking out at a cluster of tiny white buildings near the island's lighthouse. I imagined waking up on the island the following morning, joining the lighthouse keeper at the top of the tower to watch for passing dolphins while sipping hot coffee. A small yellow boat pulled in close to the headland to pick up the group and I had a strong urge to go with them, but we needed to get to Aberdaron for dinner.

When I'm out walking, I sometimes feel as though I could walk forever into the horizon and never stop. I had that feeling that day. But at the same time my stomach knew it needed to be fed and it would only be so long before blisters appeared on my heels. I have often found myself going too far without a Paula to steady me, to remind me of what might happen if we carry on. She was a trained mountain leader, after all and it was why we made such a great hiking team. She knew the importance of dinner and rest.

In the same way, my ex-husband's steady practicality often saved me from going too far when we were together. I longed just to keep going – to keep drinking, to keep partying, to keep travelling into the unknown – but he always stopped me and made sure I didn't go too far. But in the end, I resented the restrictions he placed on my freedom and I was determined to escape from him. I could have stayed safely tethered to him but I chose to break free. There was something inside me that wanted to run into the horizon and never stop.

The next morning, after breakfast at the hotel, we stopped at the bakery, *Becws Islyn*, to stock up on pies and cake for the hike ahead to Abersoch. As we left the village, I spotted a church and a graveyard spilling down to the sea and longed to go in, but we didn't have time. My list of places to come back to was steadily growing.

After leaving the wild and wuthering coastline of Aberdaron, the path took us on a detour through country roads and farm tracks, until we could see a long strand of sand below us. It was completely empty. We found out later that the mile-long Neigwl beach was entirely walkable – we just needed to time it with low tide – but we dutifully followed the detour signs inland. It was one of the many moments when I wish I'd bought the official Wales Coast Path guidebook.

But then, even though the sun shone and the birds tweeted, there was something terribly wrong with the farmland we were walking through. It was clear that the farmer didn't want anyone to be there and he (or she) had systematically removed the official Coast Path signage, locked gates, blocked hedges and anything else that would have made our way easier. It was the exact opposite of the warm Welsh welcome we'd received until now. I felt a dark presence hanging there, as though the spiritual mists of Aberdaron had forced it back to this point.

The signs became even clearer when we encountered the carcass of a sheep strewn across the path as though it had been part of some of sort of satanic ritual. Maggots and flies were crawling all over it. We knew it was illegal for any farmer in the UK to leave dead animals lying around and vowed to report it once we were away from the dark lands. But whichever way we went, we were blocked, and we ended up backtracking past the dead sheep again and onto a country road.

Paula eventually found a route that would lead us closer to Abersoch – and it was then that we found ourselves crossing a field full of young bullocks. Fifteen young bullocks who decided it would be fun to repeatedly charge us in a frisky fashion. I have never felt so vulnerable or so scared. Thankfully, Paula's quick thinking resulted in her remembering her dad's trick – clashing her walking poles together loudly in front of her to frighten them off. While she did that,

I tried to repeat calming words, but I think what came out of my mouth repeated was, "Fuck." I only had one pole with me.

That evening we reported the farmer to Gwynedd Council and DEFRA and discovered that the same farm and farmer had been reported for the same thing in 2004 when a TV news team found numerous dead cows, calves, sheep and lambs there. The farm was called Neigwl, like the beach we'd detoured from, so I looked up what the Welsh word meant: Hell's Mouth. Hell's Mouth Farm. It was nominative determinism at its finest.

It was a relief to be in the safe haven of Abersoch after our dead sheep and frisky bullock encounter. I had memories of holidaying in the town with my mother, staying at a nearby caravan park but I didn't recognise any of it. We took a rest day the next day and I discovered a town that was a live version of the Boden catalogue, filled with capable and attractive dyed-blonde mums in striped Breton T-shirts buying overpriced boho dresses and surf gear from their friends' boutiques. It was clear to me that the locals had long fled – the comparison with Welsh-speaking Aberdaron was stark.

The sub-text was a story I'd heard over and over again for years – how local Welsh people were being priced out of the housing (and business) market by wealthy 'blow-ins' from England. I'd seen it in places like the Brecon Beacons and Pembrokeshire, and now it was happening here. The pandemic only served to increase the demand for Welsh coastal properties as people realised they could live here and work online. The Abersoch I remembered had bucket-and-spade seaside shops selling trinkets made out of shells. Now it was chi-chi restaurants and wine bars with waiting lists in a town referred to as 'Cheshire-on-sea'. My mother would be turning in her grave ... or would she? She liked a bit of beach glamour and perhaps that life would have suited her better than a caravan park. *Smashing for the beach*, she'd say, pulling on a boho dress bought from the Freemans catalogue and some nice gold sandals.

How Elizabeth Pamela Mary loved to pore over her catalogues for clothing entirely unsuited for Welsh weather, never really having left the life she had with my father in first decade of their marriage – living in Kenya, as colonial civil servants. She owned filmy blouses, white skirts and strappy sandals that barely saw the light of day, except when I nicked them as a teenager to 'style up' with my eighties wardrobe. At one point, even with nearly forty years between us, we were more like girlfriends who used to shop in Chester together, selecting items in Warehouse (when it belonged to Jeff Banks) having tea and cake in Browns department store and buying something nice from Marks and Spencer for tea before catching the bus back to Wales.

A side of me liked a glamorous beachside setting too, and she was in full force as Paula and I sat having breakfast at the exclusive beach restaurant of a luxury seaside holiday park, with its spa, heated outdoor pool, boathouse and helicopter pad. We'd been allowed in by reluctant staff as they were only supposed to open for 'owners' in the park during the pandemic. It was a huge restaurant with an outdoor area with plenty of space to socially distance. For the second time, I felt unwelcome in Wales and it made me feel very sad.

The last leg of our hike took us to Criccieth, which I'd visited as a child but had no memory of its elegant Victorian frontage. It was charming, with a small castle on its main headland, a couple of tiny tearooms, an award-winning ice-cream parlour and the beautiful white art-deco-style Dylan's restaurant on the seafront.

More importantly for me, it was just under two miles away from Morfa Bychan, Black Rock Sands, where I'd stayed with my mother in a caravan park after my father died. I remembered us taking our Jack Russell, Sherry, and letting her loose on the sand there, watching her bolt away into the distance, unable to comprehend the range of her freedom. I longed to return.

Paula agreed that it would make another great rest-day short hike and we walked alongside the railway line and some country roads to get there, with, unbelievably, the sun still shining. I felt seriously blessed. It was as though the Welsh gods had collectively decided to sell my home country back to me by showing it in its best light, literally. My eyes could only see the dancing light of the sea, making everything beside it sparkle.

As soon as my feet hit the hard, rippled sands of Morfa Bychan, I felt her there. My mother. Her hand slid into mine, as it had done not long before she died, and she was smiling, laughing.

After my father died, the light inside my mother largely went out and she struggled to keep going with life in general. He had been the social lighthouse, drawing everyone to him and once he was no longer there, she disappeared into the darkness again. She would book a week or two in a caravan in Abersoch, Porthmadog or Morfa Bychan from time to time and take me with her, sometimes with one of my friends. I don't remember her socialising with anyone, just sitting alone in the caravan doing crosswords or walking on the beach with me and the dog. Maybe she was just quiet and introverted, something I was beginning to relate to now, spending most of my days on my own. I'd always understood her enforced solitude and aloneness as stemming from her grief but now I wondered if it was a state she longed for, even without me in tow. After years of pretending to be an extravert in the workplace just to keep my head above water, I had rediscovered the original me during lockdown and I drew my energy from being alone in nature. I had a feeling that I'd inherited this from my mother, whilst my father was clearly an extravert, loving a social group situation. As a couple, they balanced each other out: yin and yang.

My mother was with me now, alone, smiling beside me on the sand, and I could feel her joy. I smiled back, leaving the real world behind. Paula later told me that she could see something was happening and let me walk alone for a while. I could physically feel my mother's presence in the breeze and in the dancing light of the shallow waters. It would not be the first time I would feel it and it would not just be my mother who joined me in the wind.

In that moment, I told my mother that I was publishing my book. I told her that I had found my home again in North Wales and its true beauty had revealed itself to me. I would experience its joy just as she had. In solitude, with myself.

On the walk home I had a lightbulb moment – yes, my mum had seemed depressed after the loss of her husband, on a downward spiral, but his loss had occurred at exactly the same time as the onset of her own menopause. I suddenly saw her irritability with me, a pubescent fourteen-year-old girl, through a different lens. And one that could have been softened if she'd been offered HRT. Instead, she'd become a hermit.

Back at the hotel in Criccieth after dinner at Dylan's, I decided to go off for an hour on my own to explore the town for one last time. I was feeling the pull of solitude again, and the need to commune not just with my mother, but with my past self again. In these places I'd been a clever young girl with a crush on Kate Bush and an obsession with *Wuthering Heights*, shy and smiling, enjoying ballet classes and walking on her own with her dog. There was no unhappy marriage, no cheating, no addiction to alcohol, no toxic workplaces, no emotional turmoil – just a deep hunger for a life beyond the Welsh horizon. And all that hunger, in the end, had led me straight back to it.

On the train back south, I made the decision to return to my hometown, Holywell, to see if I could see it through the glittering lens I'd discovered in the Llŷn. I would go on a pilgrimage to Ynys Môn, Anglesey, back to the beaches where both my parents had taken me as a child. I would be by myself ... but not.

WORTHING, WEST SUSSEX
ENGLAND, JULY-AUGUST 2021

But before anything else, I had a book that I needed to publish. I'd decided that to avoid any potential backlash or trolling, I would publish under a pseudonym. I would also sanitise my story by calling the book '*Breakfast Dress*', referring to a tradition I had when holidaying alone – putting my best dress on in the mornings. Initially this practice helped to fight the demons I was dealing with overnight, but it soon became a joy in itself. Nothing sparkles more brightly than a sequin or a glittering bead in the morning sunshine. Plus I avoided any 'woman of the night' glances by wearing those things at an unexpected time. I traditionally dressed down for dinner, so it didn't look like I was 'advertising for business'.

I was still very concerned about the content of my book, partly due to the reaction of my advance readers who were split 50/50 between those that loved it and wanted to share it with all their friends and those that were worried for me, about how my dark horses would be received by strangers. Not only that, but on my second visit to Miriam, my parents were showing her pages of my book in a fire. I immediately thought that this might mean I should burn the whole idea. But Miriam told me that fire meant change, transformation, and the work I was doing on the book to rid it of its demons was doing that job. *"Write from the heart and not the ego,"* Miriam had said – I was sticking to that mantra religiously.

I briefed the designer, my friend and ex-colleague, Clare – she was someone whose creative intelligence and straight-forward thinking I valued enormously. I knew she'd have the right vision for the book. My brief was a generic *'woman finds herself on Indian beach'*. My vision contained mala beads, an icon of Ganesha and a breakfast dress, all laid out on peacock colours and dark Indian teak. *Breakfast Dress*, by Angharad Shaw. I was rather pleased with it. Angharad was the perfect name for a Welsh woman 'taken by the wind' on a Goan beach.

Clare came back to me almost immediately. "Umm, do you have another title? I'm struggling to find the right dress. Something about it isn't coming together."

I thought for a moment.

"Well, there is the original title: *Cheat Play Live*. And the image of the shell I found on the beach in San Francisco."

"You know that's it, don't you?"

Of course it was. As soon as the words were typed into a text I knew they were the right choice, even though I felt sick at the thought of the unflinchingly powerful title. I'd been working on edits to the book and on one morning's beach walk, I realised that what connected all my experiences were beaches around the world, from Wales to Turkey, Egypt to Goa. Each of the beaches would form chapters of my book and the shell image would be perfect for the cover. And now I could add a three-part structure to hold everything together, the sections entitled: *Cheat, Play* and *Live*. Editorially, the book began to fall into its natural place – only a month before the intended publication date on 14 August – my mother's birthday.

I also decided to use my own name. If the title was going to be so overtly showcasing my dark horses, then I would own it completely. No more hiding.

The choice of publication date went against everything my publishing career had ever taught me about launching a debut book. A Saturday in August was absolutely the worst time to launch anything – when everyone had already bought their beach reads and was now on holiday – but I was determined to publish it when it felt right to me. I was in control of this process and it felt crazily good. I'd also decided not to show the revised draft under its new title to anyone except Shubham. He read it while he was on board ship and he told me he loved it, that it had made him cry. He'd also felt jealous of the other men in the book, especially Luke whose name he still could not utter, but he looked beyond them all to the person whose story it was: mine.

I also decided not to try and seek representation by an agent again. I'd done it for the first draft and realised that I should never have shown that version to anyone. It was unformed, uncrafted and filled with bitterness, blame and ego; the people I showed it to said people might not react well to it. The new version was completely different but I doubted anyone would give it a second chance, seeing it as just another *Eat, Pray, Love* homage. Plus, I could see that the publishing industry was in a huge period of transition and looking for stories from writers of colour. There was no way anyone was going to pick up another story of a white, middle-aged woman finding herself on a Goan beach. And that was how it should be. I decided I would make this happen myself and in that decision, I found freedom.

I felt a huge rush of energy propelling me towards publishing the book. In our last session, Miriam had seen my father clasping his hands together in a pleading fashion and we concluded that he was willing me on (although in the darkest hours of the night I wondered if he was saying the opposite – *Stop! You don't know what you're about to unleash!*).

About two weeks before publication I put the book up for pre-order on Amazon with Clare's cover. I pressed '*share*' on a Facebook post, smiled to myself and left for my beach walk.

Shubham's ship was due to sail past Worthing on its way to the Netherlands that day and when I checked my ship-tracking app, I discovered that he was moored offshore, just behind Rampion wind farm, which was around twelve miles off the coast.

I ran to the end of the pier as my eyes picked out a shape beyond the white turbines. I knew it was him. My love. He wouldn't have a signal while out at sea, but I knew we didn't need one. We broadcasted to each other through the universe and our souls acknowledged the exchange.

I've done it! I've told the world about my book! I said in my heart.

I could see him smiling and saying, "*You have that type of talent.*"

I finally received a message from Shubham telling me he was being allowed to leave the ship on August 7. He was docked in Southampton, a train ride away from me, and he'd have exactly four hours to be with me.

Miriam smiled when I told her the news, "It's because you have finished your book," she said. "Now you are allowed to see him."

She was right – Shubham's message had come through only when I'd completed all the changes to it. She'd been right about me being left alone purposefully by the universe, to complete my project.

I walked quickly from the train station to the Queen Elizabeth dock in Southampton, furiously texting Shubham on WhatsApp. We would be with each other in under thirty minutes. After all the waiting and separation, after him contracting coronavirus, two lots of isolation and a neverending orbiting of the UK, Shubham was finally going to be standing in front of me.

"Turn your location on," he texts, so I do as he asks.

We both appear as small blue dots on the screen. His is moving quickly.

"Are you in a taxi?!" I text.

No answer.

I speed up, and his blue dot gets even faster, moving closer to mine. I turn into the bleakest industrial road I've ever seen, lined with imported cars on raised platforms. They're grey and silver Minis, and I notice that they have the Union Jack on their roofs, also in grey and silver.

There is a sound that can only be described as a seagull in great distress calling over and over in a maddening way. I realise that it's a recording to keep real seabirds from spoiling the cars. There are no visible humans around.

Our dots are even closer. I look up and see someone coming towards me at speed, a tall, dark man wearing a black and white print shirt. He is holding up his phone, as though recording me.

"It's you!" I cry as we begin to run towards each other, laughing.

We embrace and I feel the warmth of Goan sunshine through Shubham's print shirt, which is covered in Sanskrit symbols. It is a type of open-necked shirt worn in Goa that looks so out of context here in the grim industrial greyness of an English dockyard. His smile, too – filled with joy and love – feels like it doesn't belong here, but it does ... in my heart.

We hold hands and walk back towards the town, wanting to make the most of our four hours. We stop to take selfies in the shade of a tree and our smiles are cheesy.

We cross the road outside the place I have booked for lunch and laugh as a carriage drawn by two white horses goes past and then pulls up exactly where we enter the building. We both know it's the spirit of White Horse. She is no more, but her spirit lives on. She is blessing us.

Many of my friends had shared my writing journey in April 2019 and were delighted to see that I hadn't abandoned the project. A few of them knew about my dark horses and wanted to read the book to find out the juicy details. I dreaded people like my ex-husband reading it, but I braced myself for the response. I'd been as kind as I could to the people in my story and done my best to accept my agency in anything bad that had happened. I was taking responsibility and if anything, blaming myself for everything.

But in the 3am darkness, I would imagine facing a barrage of criticism about the things that I'd done. Years before, I'd written an anonymous piece for a broadsheet newspaper about using a dating site for married people and the trolling had been merciless. Half the readers had called me a whore and the other half thought the story was made up by the newspaper's editors to get attention. In the dark nights of my soul, I saw the fire my parents had been showing to Miriam, and it was not a place of rebirth or transformation – it was where I would be burned alive.

But then, when I actually pressed the button, nothing happened. Positive comments and reviews began to roll in and I breathed a sigh of relief that no one was suggesting I burned at the stake. Anything but; in fact, people said my decision to publish my story had been brave and they were impressed with the level of honesty. They said they were unable to put my book down. A significant number admitted to doing the same things as me. It made me happy that people related to it, even if our situations were very different. I heard from women and men I knew and didn't know, telling me that they were grateful I'd published my story.

Some of my ex-colleagues were expecting me to slate the toxic work environments we'd shared but I decided not to rant – I focused on how the challenging individuals I'd encountered had affected me and me alone, rather than make sweeping statements on behalf of people who may have experienced things differently. After all, there were people who flourished under those regimes so I stuck purely to my experience. Early readers said I'd been kinder than they expected to my ex-husband, ex-lovers and ex-bosses. I was pleased – Miriam's advice (or the advice of the spirits delivering messages to her) had been right.

Naïvely, I thought I would press the *'publish your book'* button on Amazon and that would be it. The book would find its readership and I could walk away, happy that I'd finally done it. But no. My debut book turned out to be the child I'd finally had by choice. I'd brought it into the world and it was my responsibility to keep it alive by whatever means and make sure it had the best start in life. Every waking moment was spent tweaking copy, emailing contacts, asking for reviews, working out how to promote and advertise it. Every day, I discovered something new I should be doing as a self-published author, having joined a few forums. It was overwhelming and it started to seriously affect my ability to get my paid work done.

This is how it feels to be an author, I thought, having spent twenty-five years on the other side of the desk, wondering why they were often angst-filled people. Before pressing the '*publish your book*' button I hadn't even know what Amazon categories, key words and chart positions were, but soon friends started commenting on mine and I started looking. I forgot that I had originally decided to publish the book to fulfil a creative urge and to help people, and I focused on the numbers on my dashboard instead. I was suddenly embarrassed that I'd only reached number 18 in 'self-help' on launch day, because if I'd known about and used all the strategies that other self-published authors had, I might have got an Amazon 'bestseller badge'. People started to ask how many copies I'd sold and I began to freak out that this had been the last thing I'd paid attention to when I launched. I'd gone in blind and now I looked like a fool in front of the whole industry.

The decision to write and publish my own book also set off a process of laying bare all my relationships with people. For the most part, this was a joyous thing, with support and encouragement from expected realms, and some unexpected sources, such as school friends and colleagues from years gone by. All sorts of people popped out of the woodwork to congratulate me, to promote the book on social media, and even to offer to try and sell the book in their cafés and shops. I was blown away by friends in the media world who, without even being asked, simply did what they could to ensure my book got the best start in life. I'll always be eternally grateful to those who showed such kindness.

But people I'd counted among my closest friends struggled to acknowledge that I'd even written a book. They hid behind embarrassingly weak excuses for why they couldn't read it and it was clear that even mentioning it was a struggle. Friends I'd been absolutely sure would support me simply went mute from the moment I revealed the cover and to this day, have never asked me about the book. It was as though they were ignoring my newborn child, a child that had quickly become a central part of my existence and there was nothing left for us to talk about. It felt like a bomb had gone off in friendships that I thought could withstand anything and they died in what seemed like an instant.

I'd already had a preview of this scenario and naïvely thought it was a one-off. Two years earlier, I'd showed my first draft to a good friend who ran a large book group. It was the version containing all my dark horses and I felt they would be safe with her. But in the summer of 2019, I discovered that they weren't safe with her at all.

I'd made myself go to an event she was hosting because she'd been feeling low and I wanted to support her. But when I arrived, in front of an assembled crowd of book-group members, she told me that she was struggling with my story because she was 'moral'. She kept saying the word over and over, getting louder and louder. "I have morals!" she cried, as the other guests began to ask questions about my book. It was breathtakingly judgemental and the last reaction I expected from a close friend.

I made my excuses and left the event early, stunned and unable to comprehend what had just happened. I walked along Regents Canal in the sunshine that day, back to my flat in Kensal Rise, ruminating on what my friend had blurted out. Was what I'd written so dreadful? It must have been. This was the reaction from someone I trusted who worked in publishing, after all. I texted my friend Elv, an editor and trained psychotherapist and one of the first people to read and support my book. She had been with me on a San Franciscan beach when I found the shell that was to change my life, featured on the cover of *Cheat Play Live*.

Elv was horrified and tried to tell me that this reaction exposed more about the person who said it than my book. But the damage was done. I put the text away into a folder on my desktop, afraid to show it to anyone else in case it elicited the same reaction.

Now, witnessing so-called close friends fall silent or make cringeworthy excuses turned a light off in my soul. Hearing them tell me all about another book they'd just chosen for their next book club was a nail in the coffin of friendship. I didn't expect worldwide adulation but was it too much to expect good friends to support me? By contrast, Shubham was telling anything that moved about my book. He was proud, especially of being in it, and he'd said he'd do all he could to make everyone read it. He is still doing it, even as I write these words, accosting unsuspecting passengers on his ship and writing the title down on a napkin.

I quickly entered a period of grief for all the friendships I'd lost or been forced to recalibrate during this process and the urge to stay solitary grew stronger. I folded in on myself, only able to cope with chatting to passing strangers and my friends on the seafront every morning. Then I'd scuttle back to my kitchen table where I worked and watch the birds feed on the food I'd put out for them and a fox run along my garden wall at the same time every evening. Thank goodness for animals – they were never disappointing.

BENLLECH, ANGLESEY
NORTH WALES, SEPTEMBER 2021

I decided it was time to embark on my second pilgrimage back to Wales, to fulfil the pact I'd made with myself on the Llŷn a few months before. I wanted to explore Anglesey, Ynys Môn, the place where my parents had taken me as a baby and a little girl. When I was six or seven, I remember sitting with my parents in the Bay Hotel in Trearddur Bay, listening to the staff tell me what a joyful, bouncing baby I'd been. But all I could think about was my mother making me go in the water at Rhosneigr in my knickers in front of a boy that morning. I'm still embarrassed about it.

I don't know why, but I chose Benllech as the place I would stay. I'm normally a west-coast girl, having noticed that I'm naturally oriented towards the west of anywhere I go, but Benllech sits on the east coast of the island. However, the entire island is situated off the north-west coast of Wales so my general orientation would no doubt be fine, I decided. I liked the look of the town, with its cafés, restaurants and shops and a big, wide beach where people took their dogs for exercise. I had a feeling I would like the place.

I booked a shepherd's hut on Air BnB and got a message from Louise the host. She offered to come and pick me up from Bangor station if I needed it. *Ah*, I thought, *there it is – the welcome in the hillside.*

She and her husband, Eric, greeted me off the bus from Bangor.

"Oh, she's a local!" Eric said in a thick North Welsh accent I hadn't heard for decades. "She's from Treffynnon!"

Treffynnon is the Welsh name of my hometown, Holywell (it means, literally, 'holy well'). It was so wonderful to hear a man speaking with an accent like my father's again. That telltale emphasis on the second syllable of every word, the elliptical sound of an 'O' in the back of the throat as he said 'local'. My hosts completely accepted me as a local, despite my posh publishing accent. (On the Llŷn, an elderly woman had commented on my pronunciation of local place names: *"It's very good for an English person!"* I'd been horrified and saddened.)

I moved into my tiny hut and was immediately delighted. As with my flat in Worthing, I found the small space comforting. I loved having only what I needed and no more. Most of my belongings were still in storage – I'd only taken some clothes and kitchenware out to help me during the lockdowns. And now, all I had was the pack on my back in my hut.

The hut sat on the piece of land adjoining Louise and Eric's large house overlooking the town, about a ten-minute walk away from the sea. It had its own balcony and wicket-fenced garden, should guests wish to bring a well-behaved dog with them (one day!).

The hut was clad inside and out with wooden panelling and had a small woodburner and wood pile to one side of the double doors. Welsh checked reversible blankets were folded neatly over two pale-blue wool-covered chairs and the bed was snugly fitted into one side of the hut, its window facing north. I decided to eat in that night and bought some salad items and alcohol-free prosecco from the nearby supermarket after an evening walk on the beach. As I packed everything away in the little fridge tucked into the galley kitchen, I felt content. I couldn't wait to start hiking the Wales Coast Path the next day.

The plan wasn't to circumnavigate the whole island – I have realised that I am not a completist, I'd rather walk the parts of a path that appeal to me and leave the rest for those that feel they need to take in less-attractive parts for the sake of saying they've 'done' it. I consulted a small guidebook I'd bought and identified a few stretches I could do from Benllech, ensuring I could get home every night. One of the essential things to know about Anglesey is the scarcity of public transport or taxis, especially on a Sunday. Louise and Eric offered to pick me up at any point if I needed it, if they were available.

The sun was shining as I walked to a local café to order a sandwich lunch for my first leg: Cemaes Bay to Amlwch. It was a Saturday and buses were running, so I knew I'd be able to get to Cemaes and back from Amlwch relatively easily. Before starting the hike, I lingered awhile among Cemaes' brightly coloured shops and houses, my mother's sister having told me the family had holidayed there. I strolled along the harbour wall and listened to the local fishermen below shouting up to friends in Welsh. It was time to begin.

To begin at the beginning, the opening lines of Welsh

writer, Dylan Thomas' *Under Milk Wood* immediately pinged into my head. I'd been mildly obsessed with Thomas' output since studying it at school and it made so much sense here, in these fishing villages with their watchful seabirds and wizened salty sea dogs, just like Captain Cat. I longed to sleep at night by the '*sloeblack, slow, black, crowblack, fishingboat-bobbing sea*' of a town like the fictional Llareggub (it spelled 'bugger all' backwards).

Coming out of Cemaes, I hiked up a steep hill behind the derelict Llanlleiana old porcelain works and the tiny stony beach lying nearby, where kayakers were pulling their neon-coloured boats in for rest and refreshment. I rounded the northernmost headland of the island and found St Patrick's Church, Eglwys Llanpadrig. It is the oldest church in Wales, having allegedly been founded by St Patrick in AD 440. Its graveyard was draped over the headland, overlooking an islet where St Patrick is said to have been shipwrecked.

I remembered the unvisited church and cemetery in Aberdaron and concluded that a grave by the sea was the best place to have one, forever looking out onto a limitless horizon, anointed by seaspray and cleansed by the wind. The church was closed because of coronavirus, but if I'd been able to go inside, I'd have found an Islamic-inspired interior. Lord Stanley of Alderly had converted to Islam after marrying a Spanish Moorish woman and in 1884, refurbished the church's interior to showcase his new faith. My guidebook told me that blue tiles and blue glazed windows lay inside; a return visit was inevitable.

I pressed on and found I had the path largely to myself. Miles would go by without anyone hiking past me, and I found it both exhilarating and slightly worrying. What if something were to go wrong? No one knew I was here – I'd forgotten to tell Louise and Eric where I was going. But then I encountered Brian, a man in his late sixties, perhaps early seventies, wearing classic birdspotting gear – army fatigues, faded cap, rucksack and hiking boots – with his binoculars slung around his neck.

As he stopped to talk to me, Brian's dogs, Skye and Patsy, scurried around his legs. Skye the sheepdog arrived at his favourite spot, between Brian's legs, with which his owner stood heroically as we spoke, feet wide apart with his hands on his hips. Patsy the labradoodle lay quietly nearby.

Brian had moved to Anglesey with his wife from the Wirral for his retirement. His wife still worked on the peninsula and commuted back and forth. Brian was learning Welsh as it was so widely spoken. I bemoaned the loss of my own language and told him I was vowing to pick it up again too.

We spoke about the joys of solo hiking and Brian said, "When you're in a couple, you don't speak to anyone else, do you? We wouldn't be having this conversation now if we were with other people."

I had never thought of it like that, but it was true. Hiking with another person effectively cut you off from anyone else, unless you or the stranger needed help. As I walked on, I took what he'd said one step further: a marriage effectively cut you off from the world because you were almost never without your partner.

I had realised this on my New Zealand honeymoon with my ex-husband. We thought it had been a brilliant idea to hire a motorhome and drive it around South Island, but what it did was cut us off even more from any potential human interaction. All we managed was the odd chat with a petrol station attendant or waiter, which we engaged in after our solitary confinement in the motorhome like hungry dogs on a bone.

By far the best thing about any of our holidays were the other people we'd met – in 2005 in Namibia, we'd hired a 4X4 and gave lifts to any locals we saw walking along the roads in the heat (there was no public transport system). They spoke khoisan with all the clicking sounds we'd heard on the radio there, and we communicated with hand signals. We all laughed when the car bumped over something and we hit our heads on the roof and my ex offered cigarettes which were gratefully received (only partially smoked by our guests and kept for later). Some things are universal.

These were the memories we took home with us, along with the animals we'd seen at the waterholes. Where else would you get to pick up a Himba woman with her hair braided in rich red cornrows, and take her to find her baby's things that were placed under a random bush on the side of the road? The baby was called Gregory and had beautiful large brown eyes. I still think about him and wonder how his life panned out, as I do with Chris the student, who told us (in English) that he was going to university in Europe.

I continued on my way towards Porth Wen and its abandoned brickworks. Its tall chimneys and beehive kilns still studded the cove and provided a platform for a lunch stop for weary hikers. However, it was a fair detour down from the coast path so I decided to lunch on a grassy slope high above the brickworks and take in the view. Brian had told me that during the pandemic, families had illegally camped on the brickworks because of its flat surface near the cove. All over the island, I heard stories about how staycationers had flooded there in their thousands, trying to find some space and freedom during the various lockdowns.

As I walked, finding my own space and freedom, thoughts of the friendships I'd lost kept bursting unbidden into my mind. I couldn't shake the disappointment and the grief I was experiencing, and that I had caused this massive exposure of all my relationships by publishing my book. I'd be willing to bet that nothing exposes the people who do and don't have your back more than publishing a book. It's clear as day who is supporting you and who isn't and you can't help measuring it in the 'data' of social-media reactions, posts, shares, ratings and reviews.

I mentally trawled through the backhistories with friends I'd lost and found three distinct threads running through all of them: being judged for something I'd done, being unsupported when a good thing happened, and the worst of all for me – being competed with. Those three things were huge triggers for me; in essence, these people were great friends when the chips were down but nowhere to be seen when the chips were up. I had previously only viewed each remembered incident as isolated but now they emerged as a string of red flags, like bunting. I had a name for people like this: foul-weather friends. I'd cut off contact with a family member for the same reasons and I knew the signs.

I consulted Sudhir about it and he texted back: '*In your heart don't think bad about them. Understand that they are like that and they have to learn and grow. Just forgive. In my opinion this is the best strategy.*'

I knew it was the best strategy, but I was finding it really hard to move past it all and remember that these were good people who'd just let their own dark horses get the better of them. I was holding on to anger and resentment, and as the old saying went, it was like drinking poison yourself and expecting the other person to die. As my first day of hiking came to a close, I ruminated darkly on it all, throwing my 'relationship' with Luke into my huge bag of worries along with everything else.

I was heading into my final destination, Amlwch, along a rough track beside a playground. It was the grimmest part of my hike that day, entering the town through the pebble-dashed estates surrounding it. Suddenly, a tiny bird flew directly across my path and sat on a bush, a weed with yellow flowers, swaying gently in the wind. I expected him to fly off at any moment, scared of my presence, but instead he simply sat there. His eyes appeared to be closing, as though he was sleepy. He had fluffy speckled beige feathers, but underneath, a black and yellow chevroned tail stuck out.

It was one of the most beautiful things I'd ever seen in nature. I got closer with my phone and began to video him, a bird I later found out was a young goldfinch. He still didn't move – apparently they're naïve about their proximity to danger. I related hard – I never seemed to be able to sense red flags in the moment – they only appeared to me later, when I could see a pattern emerging. And once that pattern was seen, not only was it too late but I could never unsee it.

I didn't want to become one of those people who were distrustful and suspicious of everyone they met but I needed to protect myself a little. I decided that one of the ways I could do that was by withholding some of the information I would usually share about what I was doing. If I shared too much, especially on social media, it always elicited a round of comments I didn't feel comfortable with: people telling me I was lucky or that they were jealous, or asking me questions so that they could copy or compete with whatever I was doing. I decided I wouldn't 'check in' everywhere or tell anyone how many miles I'd walked, as I would normally do. I'd tell them

I'd met a goldfinch that day and that would be enough. I was so used to broadcasting everything: in person, on social media and now in my book; I wondered if my ego had taken it all too far and needed to retrench in silence for a while.

The goldfinch was clearly unfazed by my presence and so I decided to stay with him for a while. I thought he might be unwell, but apparently these birds are dozy when they are growing – probably because their bodies are busy making their extraordinary plumage. I felt grateful that I'd stopped to stand with him for a while – with no planned time to get back to Benllech, I could take my time and arrive back at my shepherd hut just before sundown. There were buses every hour on a Saturday so I'd be fine. This moment, even after all the miles of walking and the spectacular coastline I'd witnessed, was easily the highlight of the day. A close second was the impromptu fish-and-chip supper I took back to the hut from Finney's in Benllech.

I spoke to Shubham that night from the hut – his ship was somewhere off the coast of Scotland, en route to the Shetlands. I'd been teaching him how to say the longest place name in the world, as taught to me by my father on child-hood trips to Anglesey. He could say *Llanfairpwllgwyn* fairly passably but was struggling with the double L sound where the tongue flattens between your back teeth and you breathe out with lips pulled open to the sides. Instead of '*gyllgogery*', Shubham said '*gishgogerish*' and I'll say it like that forever in my head now. I probably sounded the same when I said something in Konkani. '*Kitay zale tuca?*' was one of only a handful of phrases he'd taught me, but there was a distinct tonality to the question – *What happened to you?* – that I couldn't quite get.

Shubham asked me if I'd smiled that day and if I'd eaten

proper food and I had to force down an irritated response. *Why do I have to smile? Why does he have to police my food intake?* I thought, not realising that he was asking from a place of love and care for my wellbeing. I told him I was struggling to smile because I was going over and over the events of the past few months and I told him what Sudhir had said about being compassionate and forgiving to my lost friends.

"I have been saying the same thing and you have not been listening!"

It was true. Shubham had been reminding me that these were my friends who had been good to me in the past. I knew that – that's why the current situation hurt so much. I tended to listen to Sudhir because he was older and wiser, but here was my young old soul, telling the truth I needed to hear.

"It is not good for you, thinking these things, Lisann. I want to see you smile again. No – not that fake one. A real one, with the holes in your cheeks."

For a twenty-six-year-old, Shubham could read me extremely well.

The next day, a Sunday, I managed to get an early bus back up to Amlwch to hike the coast back to Benllech, knowing I'd struggle to get any buses later in the day. I had breakfast at The Quays – a family run café I'd stopped in the evening before and planned to come back to because they were friendly.

This hike took me to Point Lynas, a telegraph station with a lighthouse positioned on a rocky headland, the Llaneilian promontory. The path to it was a short detour off the main route and I thought about not doing it, but something was calling me there. I wanted to see what was at the end.

The cluster of buildings at the end of the headland were castellated and bright white in the sunshine. I'd had some rain on my way there and had finally got some use out of the waterproofs I'd carried everywhere. *If Wales carries on being this sunny,* I thought, *it'll have to rebrand itself.*

There, I found a National Coastwatch station, a cabin just in front of the lighthouse. The cabin had the greatest view so far – the Great Orme at Llandudno to the east, Amlwch to the west and the islands of East Mouse and Middle Mouse (the latter being the northernmost point of Wales). As I walked to the edge of the land, I saw a man in uniform scurrying alongside another man in fatigues with binoculars. Another Brian! I would ask him what he'd seen that day – I always ask these sorts of people what they've seen. Birdwatchers by the sea in Worthing were always full of information.

I approached the two men. They'd spotted a pod of Risso's dolphins – a species I'd never heard of, known for their bulbous heads and narrow tails. The 'birdwatcher' – Dr Richard Arnold, a former zoology professor from Bangor University – had come to Lynas specifically to see these dolphins, who were known to pass the point regularly. He looked beatific in his excitement of the prospect and lent me his binoculars so I could see them too. I briefly wondered if we should be sharing them during these corona times but decided the risk was worth it.

"I'm a poor man's David Attenborough," Dr Arnold said, his eyes wrinkling into a smile. He proudly told me he'd been responsible for setting up the RSPB reserve at South Stack near Holyhead on the island.

As we looked out to sea, a rainbow appeared above the ocean. It was the kind of Disney-esque phenomenon that might happen in Agonda – a sign from the universe that you'd connected with its light and magic. I was used to it manifesting in India but not here, in Wales. Magic had never happened to me here. But the goldfinch had alerted me to the fact that something from another realm might be accompanying me on the coastal path. Perhaps on the Llŷn too.

Dr Arnold and I talked about hiking and wildlife and agreed that the best way to experience it was hiking solo. If I'd been with someone else, this portal into a magical world of dolphins and rainbows would never had opened. I would never have approached him to ask what was happening, I would never have seen the dolphins and perhaps never even lingered long enough to see the rainbow. I always want to linger long enough. Longer, if possible.

As I left, Dr Arnold said, "You're a kindred spirit."

I took that as a compliment.

Back in Benllech, wondering if Wales had undergone a weather transplant, I was brought back to earth with a bump as heavy rain and high winds raged outside the hut for one whole day, forcing me to rest inside. Having ventured out to the supermarket, I stocked up on supplies and for the first time, I lit a fire in my woodburner stove, consulting friends on Twitter on how to do it properly. I couldn't believe I'd never lit a fire before – I'd always been the person watching someone else do it.

The hut was warm in minutes and I wrapped myself in the cross-checked woollen blanket with my laptop on my knee. I don't think I've ever felt so cosy. My mind returned to the hut I'd shared with Luke in Northumberland, the most romantic place I thought I'd ever been to. He'd lit a fire there, even though it made the hut too warm, and I'd been delighted with the idea of a man setting up camp for me, his lady. But now it struck me that true romance was being with myself in a cosy hut, in front of a fire I'd lit with my own hands, with food I'd made in a tiny kitchen, with nowhere to go except a comfortable bed at the end of the day. Alone.

That evening, after the rain abated, I took myself down to the beach where dog-owners looked more relieved to be outside than their pets.

I walked as far as the St David's rocks at the most easterly part of the beach and peeked round at Red Wharf Bay. I knew I had visited there as a child with my parents. The song of my childhood was playing on repeat in my head and I knew it wouldn't stop until I'd been there. I would go the next morning.

———

As I round the coast from Benllech into Red Wharf Bay, I spy the reed-filled sands from the muddy forest path I'm walking on. The tide is out and the sands are riven with tiny estuarine tributaries. In one there is a small boat with a bright blue sail folded into it, listing to one side.

Now standing in the bay behind the boat, I listen to the wind blowing through the reeds. As ever, when standing at water level at low tide, I imagine the sea suddenly rushing in and taking me away with her. Part of me wants her to. Part of me wants to get into the boat and sail away forever.

I remember paddling into the shallows and feeling my small feet sinking into the sands. I remember being among the reeds and feeling my dad's hand holding mine. I remember saying the words 'Red Wharf Bay' and not knowing what they meant. What was a wharf? It sounded like 'dwarf' to me, like something out of a fairytale. Red Dwarf Bay.

I continue walking along duckboard bridges with wild flowers on either side and an old stone sea wall that runs all the way to the beach at Llanddona. It is another magnificent, wide, empty beach.

As I follow the path inland through woodland, I come across a series of domed huts, like Hobbit houses in the Shire, and I meet a woman I'd seen on the other side of the bay, walking her dog. She beckons me over...

The woman, silver-haired like me and in her late fifties, offers me a cup of tea, which her husband proceeds to make inside the modern split-level hut behind her. He has shoulder-length grey hair and a surf-dude smile.

"We live here most of the time," she says, showing me round. "We bought the shell and we've added everything ourselves. We love it here."

It shows on their faces. It is a tiny home and I know what that means – existing only with what you need. Nothing more. I long for the same thing.

I ask them why there is a stuffed owl stationed above their door.

"To keep away mice," they say in unison.

Living in a fairytale house tucked into a wood near the sea has to have some drawbacks.

––––––––––

Later that day, I made it to Penmon Point, with its humbug-striped, black-and-white lighthouse set on the rocks between the headland and Puffin Island, at the north-eastern end of the Menai Strait. The sun was still shining, and I could see the Great Orme at Llandudno, and now the mountains of Snowdonia on the other side. With immense gratitude, I found the Pilot House Café open and bought myself an ice cream before walking to the edge of the rocks and seeing a brown seal's head bobbing in and out of the waves. He would be heading to Point Lynas in the trail of the Risso's dolphins, no doubt. The Coastwatch guard had said seals were regular passers-by.

I could imagine myself driving out to this point with a dog in the seat next to me, pulling up and ordering tea and cake and watching seals. I could imagine myself living here, perhaps in Llanddona in a Hobbit home or in a small cottage in Benllech. The place had quietly begun calling itself home in my heart.

HOLYWELL, FLINTSHIRE
NORTH WALES, SEPTEMBER 2021

I'D PUT OFF MY TRIP BACK TO HOLYWELL, TREFFYNNON, for two more days because I knew it was going to break this spell. I knew I was going to have to confront uncomfortable memories of my teenage years, the grimness of life after my dad died when I was only ten years old. My mother chose to become a hermit, moving us to a tiny damp bungalow on top of a hill above the town. I'd roamed the moorland up there wishing I could be swept away from it all by a mysterious stranger. He bore a passing resemblance to Heathcliff, in my mind, and I was a Kate Bush-obsessed Cathy.

My teenage years coincided with a period of struggle in North Wales, with unemployment at record levels and people haunted by lack of money and to my grief-filled eyes, a lack of joy. By the time I was twenty I'd had a series of depressed episodes and tried to take my own life with an overdose. It had been a cry for help but no one bothered answering – they had their own issues to deal with. A silence descended around what I'd done and everyone just carried on as normal.

By the time I went to university at twenty-two I couldn't
wait to get away from North Wales. I made every excuse not
to go home, even though my mum was clearly struggling in
the early stages of dementia. Maybe I didn't want to go home
because I realised what was happening and didn't want to
see it. Christmases became a guerrilla event where I would
turn up for as few days as possible, saying I needed to get
back on the 27th, as soon as the trains were running.

In reality, I went back to an empty university hall and
stayed there on my own, just glad to be in a warm, dry room
with no trace of sadness in it. Over the next decade, I would
use work as an excuse to go back down south, or a trip to my
boyfriend's family in Scotland. My mum died when I was
thirty-two and for the subsequent twenty-plus years, I rarely
returned.

I knew that the town had undergone a significant amount
of regeneration in the last few years, with local traders and
town councillors (my dad had been one in the '60s and '70s)
making huge efforts to breathe new life into it. In 2019,
Holywell had been awarded a Welsh Government grant of
almost £500,000 and had started to take pride in itself again.
It even had a community museum – my dad would have
loved that.

Holywell had once been a hive of activity, the place that
supplied the water and manpower serving the factories and
mills in the nearby Greenfield Valley in the 18th century,
producing copper, brass and cotton. My father's unpublished
memoir, *Between the Fires*, detailed some of its legacy, with
the now-defunct railway line still in operation when he was a
child between the two World Wars.

His story is filled with a cast of characters that wouldn't
be out of place in a Dylan Thomas story, complete with a

blind water carrier, Joey Barker, whose donkey pulled around a barrel on wheels, selling water at a penny a bucket. Joey had an assistant – a young boy – but if he wasn't available, the donkey knew when the barrel needed a refill and would walk back to the pump with Joey holding on at the rear. My father also described the town barber, who would excuse himself in the middle of a haircut and go upstairs with his son for a cup of tea and a heated discussion on a topic such as religion. Customers would be seen sitting in the chair for ten minutes with half a haircut, awaiting his return.

I wanted to see this Holywell, the one my father had described so lovingly, using Welsh phrases here and there in the dialogue. I'd never heard him say one word of Welsh – I was more likely to hear Swahili being uttered in our house – but here was the evidence that he'd been brought up speaking it, spending all his summers in the heart of Snowdonia.

Finally, my time was up on Anglesey – the shepherd's hut had been booked by someone else and I had no choice but to decamp to my next Air BnB (I'd been paying for both for two nights, so great was my need to stay on the island). I'd decided to stay in Ffynnongroyw ('pure well') – a place that had barely registered with me in my whole twenty-two years in North Wales, but it sat next to the Dee Estuary coastal path, just south of my hometown. It consisted of a row of terraced stone cottages, which once housed the workers from the now-closed Point of Ayr colliery, backed by woodland. I discovered a circular trail behind the place I was staying – an old granary; the whole area was probably crisscrossed with paths I'd had no idea about as a teenage girl. But now, because I'd cut my time down, I had no time to explore them. *Next time.*

I met with my cousin, Jason, and his family and after a pub lunch nearby, he offered to drive me round the old places, taking in my old family homes, including the bungalow on the hill. Things had changed slightly because of the developments around the North Wales Expressway, which didn't exist when I lived there. The area around the bungalow had been spruced up with newly planted trees and bushes, obscuring the wily, windy moor where the Maes Cynfaen estate sat, and where I did my Catherine Earnshaw impression.

Inside the estate where I'd spent my teenage years with my mother, it was in fact more grim than I remembered. The place was neglected and unloved, and now filled with cars that didn't fit into its tiny potholed roads and driveways. I needed to get out and Jason sensed it – three-point-turning out of there as fast as he could.

That night, I met my oldest friend, Coreen, in the hotel I'd worked in around the time I tried to take my life – the Stamford Gate. I wanted to overwrite those times and make happy ones instead. Coreen was the perfect person to help me do that. I'd known her since I was three and she was one of the kindest souls I'd ever encountered. She'd visited my deteriorating mother every week when I'd been avoiding her down south – unprompted and unasked. This was the stuff of real friendship.

Coreen was an only child and had recently lost her father, so now we were both orphans in the world. Coreen had messaged me when she was reading my book to say that it had brought her to tears – triggered by our girlish memories. I'd been at her house the night my dad died in a hospice. Her parents must have known why I was there and the rest of the family had gone to visit him.

"I'm always here for you. You're my sister," Coreen said, bringing me to tears, her blue eyes glistening behind her round glasses.

It was one of those friendships that didn't require constant checking in. She was simply there whenever I needed her. She didn't mark me out of ten for the gestures I made or engage in any tit-for-tat or competitive behaviour. She didn't judge me for the decisions I'd made in life, good or bad. She simply stood beside me wherever I was in the world, whether the chips were up or down, and said, "I've got you."

We agreed to be official sisters from that moment on. I needed one just as much as she did, having become estranged from my own.

The next day, the sun shone brightly again as I was picked up at the granary by Karen, a primary school friend, and whisked off to something else that didn't exist on Brynford Hill when I lived there: Holywell Pet Cemetery. It made us laugh that as teenage girls we'd hung out with metalhead boys in the cemetery by our primary school. Now here we were in our fifties, having a nice cup of tea and eggs on toast next to another graveyard.

Karen owned The Flower Bowl – a florists opposite my dad's old shop, still called 'Wilf Edwards's' by some of the older locals. It had been a shop of two halves: a newsagents' on one side and a 'card cabin' on the other. Now it was a trendy coffee shop called Marmalade.

Karen was one of those people who came out of the woodwork to suddenly champion my book and she ordered

copies for the shop to sell at a special price to locals. I was so
happy that my book would be sold in a shop opposite my
dad's. There's the universe for you.

Karen, like Coreen, had kindness stamped through her
very core and I could hear it in her throaty laugh. Funny, all
three of us were childfree-by-choice. I wondered if there was
something in the (holy) water in Holywell. The town was so
socially conservative in lots of ways but here were a band of
independent women who weren't following the normal
tracks. Here was part of my DNA, and strong independent
women were a strong thread in my hometown.

Treffynnon is a place of pilgrimage, known as the
'Lourdes of Wales'. St Winefride's Well, a natural spring, lies
at the foot of a limestone escarpment in the town beside the
Well Hill road. St Winefride was a 12th-century virgin
martyr who was beheaded by a local prince, Caradoc, for
spurning his advances. The spring allegedly appeared where
her head fell and she was later restored to life by St Beuno,
her uncle. In all my time living in North Wales, I'd never
actually visited the well, which was hugely popular. (All my
Catholic action as a girl took place at the friary in Pantasaph,
up on the hill near my home in Brynford, another pilgrimage
spot with a life-size crucifixion scene.) I felt I owed Winefride a visit to pay my respects.

The well wasn't wildly exciting itself, a small green pool
housed in a stone cloister, but the park beyond it was.
Turning off the Well Hill road, I found the main woodland
path through the old Greenfield Valley mill buildings, newly
landscaped with a seventy acre nature park, museum,
ancient abbey and five reservoirs. None of this had been here
when I was a girl – it had been a wasteland, to my young
eyes. The old Victorian school house there, Spring Gardens,

had been mentioned in my father's memoir, but I'd had no idea it had been restored. He'd attended from the age of three and his teacher was a Miss Parry. I touched the grey stone of the building and wondered if his little hand had been in the same place, if his small feet had pattered around the perimeter of the school where I now walked in the sunshine.

I continued walking down to Basingwerk – the ruins of Holywell's 12th-century Cistercian Abbey. Again, this was a place that barely figured in my girlhood. It was the name of the upper part of Holywell High School and that was all I knew. I was vaguely aware of the ruins growing up but had never visited them. As I stopped to take pictures, a rainbow appeared above the ruins. A mother with two young children were playing among the stones. "Look!" I said, pointing at the rainbow.

"Wow!" both children said in unison, running towards the arc with their hands outstretched as their mother and I exchanged a smile.

Outside the visitor centre, I saw an information board depicting a trail: the North Wales Pilgrim's Way. My finger traced the route on the board. It started right where I was standing at Basingwerk, took in Pantasaph Friary, the church I'd frequented as a child, and passed through St Asaph, where I was born. The route had been developed in 2011 and used old and new paths to reconstruct the passage of pilgrims across North Wales to Aberdaron on the Llŷn and the island I'd seen off the coast there: Bardsey (Ynys Enlli). Now it was a long-distance walk, otherwise known as the Welsh Camino.

I couldn't believe that I'd been an unwitting pilgrim, managing to complete half this route without even knowing I was on it. And yet I'd felt its pull. I'd felt a spiritual energy in

Aberdaron and longed to go back and visit the seaside church and graveyard I hadn't had time to visit months earlier.

Looking it up later, I discovered that the church at Aberdaron was St Hywyn's, the last stopping point for pilgrims on their way to Bardsey Island. Known as the 'Cathedral of Llŷn', it was the meeting point of two medieval pilgrim routes along the north and south coasts of the peninsula. It was there that pilgrims waited and prepared themselves for the short but dangerous crossing to Bardsey Island.

If ever there was a place that calling me, that island was it.

WORTHING, WEST SUSSEX
ENGLAND, OCTOBER 2021–FEBRUARY 2022

DESPITE THE BEST EFFORTS OF MY HRT PATCH, I continued to ruminate darkly on my book and the impact publishing it had had on my peace of mind. I almost began to regret that I'd done it – this unexpected life laundry had been a total shock. I had also not foreseen the extent to which I would track the book's progress. As a trade publisher, I'd never even looked at Amazon charts or categories, but suddenly they were everything. It took all my strength not to keep pressing the refresh button on my publishing dashboard. I knew what I was doing: I was checking to see that my baby was still alive.

As Christmas approached, I folded further into myself and focused on work, piling up my schedule so that I wouldn't have too much time to think about my book or the friendships I'd lost because of it.

I would bump into Miriam regularly on the seafront when I snuck out in the mornings. She always appeared when I needed her positive sparkling energy. She was moving out of the seafront house she'd shared with her partner and into a house on the other side of Worthing. She had her own dark horses to deal with but she always seemed to find time to talk through mine. She did her best to make me feel better about everything that was going on and suggested I meditated every day to regain my peace of mind.

I hadn't stepped on the yoga mat for months. I hadn't completed a single asana, breath sequence or meditative moment since the publication of my book. I didn't have enough peace of mind to settle to that, whereas before, I'd done at least thirty minutes every day. I knew it was the solution to my current situation but I couldn't seem to find the time to do it, once I'd done my work, and wasted time twiddling around with book promotion and relentlessly pressing the refresh button. In the midst of it all, my lockdown yoga students contacted me to see if I would be teaching again through the winter. I said I would think about it, but I knew I just didn't have the emotional or spiritual capacity for it.

The Cinderella-after-the-ball feeling after self-publishing was very real. I could only exist on goodwill from friends and ex-colleagues for so long. There was a 'now what?' feeling plaguing me day after day, and it wouldn't be silenced unless I tweaked something or made a tiny bit of promotion happen. In our regular daily video calls, when he could get a signal in harbour, Shubham would tell me to just stop thinking about it – just let my book be and get on with my other work. *Easier said than done, Shubs.*

Then Sudhir announced a new online course that would be on offer from December 2021 – a 40-hour Emotional Empowerment course based on the study of the Vedic text, the *Bhagavad Gita*. Students had a year to complete it.

Sudhir had left Sampoorna and set up his own yoga school operating out of North Goa. I'd completed his advanced pranayama (breathing practice), meditation and yoga philosophy courses in one hit during the summer of 2020 and found I'd become increasingly interested in the theory behind the yoga class. Once I found out from him that the poses were purely intended as a way of making your body more comfortable during long periods of meditation, I'd begun to lose interest in them. They were a small part of a very big whole – it was just that the Western world had become fixated on being able to do them gymnastically and treated them as a workout. As Sudhir said, they were very much the opposite: "*They're a 'work-in'*," he liked to say.

When I first met him, I'd been a publishing director for a number of years and had my eye on a managing-director role. I told him that I was caught in a cycle of ambition in my publishing career – I was obsessed with climbing higher and higher, with achieving the next rung on the ladder. I described it as always trying to be the brightest light on the Christmas tree and not being content to be a regular light bulb. It was making me really unhappy. Why did I need it so much?

What Sudhir said had helped to direct me on a new path. He told me that the ambition I'd mentioned was one of the three gateways to hell in the *Bhagavad Gita. 'You have to understand that you are already shining brightly. You are enough,'* he'd said. *'You don't need to prove anything or be better than anyone else.'* That conversation had been enough to set me on a path to freedom through freelancing.

Over Christmas 2021, I read the *Gita* – the story of a young man, Arjuna, on the morning of a battle, being counselled by his teacher, Krishna. The story is a metaphor for the emotional battle within Arjuna, whilst Krishna represents the universe in human form. According to Krishna, the three gateways to hell are lust, greed and anger. An intense desire (or lust) for something leads to greed as you find yourself wanting more of something by any means. Lust and greed then turn into anger when you are not able to get what you want. All three destroy your peace of mind and lead to self-destruction.

So. Many. Bells. Ringing.

The central message of the *Gita* is to act or work with no expectation of personal gain or reward:

"Those who are motivated only by desire for the fruits of action are miserable, for they are constantly anxious about the results of what they do."
Bhagavad Gita, 2. 47.

This. This was the key to resetting my brain after the publication of my book. It was to remember why I'd done it in the first place – to help others. I'd let my ego flood into the equation and had become too attached to the results. Because I'd occupied a senior position in the industry I felt as though my book's performance was on show and had to be good, whereas in reality, probably no one but me ended up looking or caring. I was self-destructing for no reason.

Everyone, almost without exception, asked me about how many copies I'd sold. I wanted to answer with how many people had messaged me to say how much they'd related to my story, but I knew it would fall on deaf ears. For some reason, people, whether they are readers or not, view publishing a book as a money-making scheme and a route to fame. Authors regularly wait for years, sometimes decades, until they get an agent or a book deal from a publisher. Self-publishing is seen as a failure because the book is not endorsed or validated by the corporate world. Now, standing outside of it all, managing my own business, I could see the truth: self-publishing is personal ownership, creative control and freedom. Somewhere along the line I'd forgotten that.

Most debut authors feel the same angst around their books as self-published ones, but at least we are in control of our child's destiny. We can play a longer game, rather than the three-month window afforded to a new trade title, after which, its destiny is decided. Hasn't sold enough? Move it off the frontlist to the midlist, and eventually the backlist, where it will barely get any promotional support.

After the *Gita*'s revelation, I knew what I had to do. I needed to redefine what success meant for me. My goal was to reach people who might be stuck in unhappy marriages, toxic jobs or a cycle of addiction and let them know through my story that they had options. It was to reach as many people as possible, not to make as much money as possible. It was to write, edit and publish a book myself and not be beholden to the corporate world to validate it for me. I wanted it to be the best it could be, as a piece of creativity; something I could be happy with as a legacy that would live beyond me.

Firstly, I decided to stop taking part in the publishing industry conversation on social media because it was only becoming a source of angst. I'd left the corporate world behind for a reason, so why was I immersing myself in the world of book deals and bestsellers every day, punctuated by the cries of authors who had or hadn't achieved either? It was only making everything worse.

Secondly, Amazon had a promotional mechanism by which authors could offer their ebook for free across five days in every 90-day cycle so I decided to do it. If the real goal for me was getting books into readers' hands and helping others, then surely this was the way to do it.

As a rule, I'd avoided free things as a consumer all my life, suspicious of the motive behind the 'seller' and the quality of the product I was getting. I had to back quickly out of all those thoughts as I promoted my free days, which were possibly my most rewarding since I'd published. People were grateful for a free story and it hit the mark for those who needed to hear its message. It was the best moment of my publishing journey by far.

In February, on a cold but sunny morning, I met a man sitting in one of the seafront shelters, with a sign up next to him offering passers-by a chat or a listening ear. I'd seen him several times before and wondered who might stop for his services in full view of promenaders. He was wearing a knitted coat and hat, from which his long grey wispy hair protruded. It occurred to me that he wouldn't look out of place in the northern mountains of India.

His sign said:

Welcome to Bram's 'Chat room'
where you can 'drop in' for a chat while passing by...
Lost a spouse, a partner, a close relative recently?
Tired, lonely, depressed?
Do you have joyful news to share?
Then STOP!

I told him that I admired what he was doing and asked if many people took him up on his offer.

"It's like fishing," Bram said, his ice-blue eyes twinkling. "I can sit here for hours and then one person will stop for a chat and make it all worthwhile."

Bram's accent was Welsh – from South Wales – and I soon discovered he was from Neath.

"I'm from North Wales! Holywell!" I said gleefully.

How wonderful to find a fellow countryman here by the sea in Sussex, especially one who was doing something so worthwhile. He asked me what I thought of his signage and I offered to help him with it, mentioning that I was an editor, writer and publisher by trade. Of course, I mentioned my book. My ego was still in charge of that one.

"Oh! Did you publish it as a commercial thing or for other reasons?"

There it was – the only time someone didn't immediately assume that publishing my book was purely a money-making scheme (which, by the way, it largely isn't, for anyone – if I wanted to make money, I'd be writing crime or romance fiction series').

"I'm like you. I want to help people who have experienced grief and tried to numb the pain by various means, including alcohol. If I can fish for one person, and help them, it'll be worth it."

I went back to my kitchen-table desk filled with the spirit of Bram, a person who gave up hours of his time to just sit and wait for one person whom he might help. No expectation of personal gain or reward, and no ego demanding that he be seen as some sort of saviour.

I wanted to Be More Bram in every way possible.

AGONDA, SOUTH GOA
INDIA, MARCH 2022

It's 7.30am and I am stumbling, drunk with joy, onto the beach to find my dogs. A red collar on jet-black fur. Sweet-pea! She is terrorising the family of pigs (new chicas!) that are living behind the Red House. The piglets are huddling together in fear under the huts on the beach, their pale pink trotters placed neatly together, like tiny ballerinas on pointe.

Sweetpea nods her head in recognition and comes closer. Oh my! She has white hair and whiskers all over her face and her eyes are rheumy red. She looks thin. Are you ok, my Sweetie?

I play a quick game of 'dog or log', something I played when I was here last. Is that Zimbo or a piece of driftwood I see lying in the sand?

A little head rises from the hole he's dug to access the cool, moist sand underneath. It's Zimbo, followed by Sanjo – both a little whiter around the face. How did they all age so much in two years?

Then I remember – I'm a little whiter too. The last time they saw me I was still growing out my silver hair.

I make my way into Simrose and Dinesh is there, smiling.
I'm unsure about hugging anyone after my flight, but Dinesh
gives me a brotherly hug. I'm home at last.

Finally, after checking daily to see if the situation would
change, India began to open its doors to international travellers. We were only allowed a 30-day visa (which we had to
obtain in person) but they dropped all formal testing proce-
dures on either side and let UK tourists travel if they either
had proof of three Covid vaccinations or a negative PCR test
72 hours before flying.

I had been volunteering for the NHS in Worthing during
the pandemic, working as a marshall at a local surgery where
queues of people came for their first, second and third jabs. It
had got me away from my desk and more importantly, away
from my ego, which was still obsessing over my situation. I
saw the elderly and the clinically vulnerable struggling to
come in for their jabs and it told my ego to sit back down and
shut up. These were people with real problems.

Now that the booster programme had done its job, the
UK ended all its restrictions on the day I flew to India –
February 24th – the second so-called 'Freedom Day'.
Shubham was home from his ship and waiting for me at the
other end. We'd been counting the days down and now, in
approximately nine hours, I would see his actual face.

I spotted him amidst the sea of taxi drivers in white calling, "Ma'am! Ma'am!" He was on the phone, frowning. This
was not the welcome I'd imagined.

He was speaking to his friend the taxi driver who was
circling around outside, waiting for a parking space. They'd

waited a long time for me and the place was chaotic at the best of times, but finally, my hand was in Shubham's in the back of the car and we were grinning madly at each other.

It was 5.30am. I lost my jetlagged self in listening to Shubham chat happily to his friend in Konkani while I took in all the sights of the towns we passed through: Margao, Chinchinim, Cuncolim, Canaguinim. I repeated the names quietly to myself, like a mantra. The chai shops were already open and people were making their way to work on foot, in tuktuks and small cars. The colourful lorries from neighbouring states rattled round on the roads causing more hair-raising overtaking moments on bends in the road. Shubham told me that they are covered – literally in bells and whistles – to alert drivers to their presence, as well as to make an aesthetic statement.

What I wasn't expecting was the beauty of the country-side at that time in the morning, filled with a low-lying mist that I'd seen in Cola over the paddy fields two years before. It now rested over the fields and wetlands where water buffaloes stood with egrets balancing on their backs.

"Agonda!" I shouted, when we turned into the road to the village, passing the women who were laying out their fresh fruit and vegetables on tables.

Marshall and Saluzhina were up and about as we pulled up outside the Red House, making the most of the cool of the morning to get their chores done. I moved into my rooms quickly and almost ran to the beach while Shubham went home to Palolem for a few hours.

It was immediately apparent that a lot had changed in Agonda since I was last there. Just as the UK tourists had staycationed at home, so had the Indian ones. Dinesh told me that social media had had a huge impact on Indian tourism in the area, and where Agonda used to be a place where Indians rarely went, it was now 'on the map' and more importantly, on Instagram. People came for shorter visits and required more activities to do while they were here, so Simrose was constantly turning around its rooms and huts while the beach was filled with double the number of boats and kayaks.

I found Nitesh near his boat that evening, talking to some Indian customers. He confirmed everything that Dinesh had told me. Whereas just before the pandemic, Agonda tourism had been suffering, now everywhere was booming with stay-cationers from nearby Mumbai and Karnataka. He was taking his boat out for two dolphin trips per day.

The next morning, at 7am, Nitesh showed me how the river at the far end of the beach, where his family had lived all their lives, had changed shape due to a recent cyclone. We witnessed a queue of fishermen, fluffy nets stored safely in their boats, waiting patiently for high tide to come and help them wind their way round the new river channel that curved between two new banks of sand. The mornings were still cool so they were clad in an array of hoodies and woollen hats in blue, yellow and red. Some were already standing thigh-deep in the water, ready to start pushing the boats round. Nitesh left me to wade in and help them bring the boats in when the tide was high enough.

As I walked back to the Red House, the young man on the mahogany horse rode past, trailing three brave beach dogs behind him. He skidded to a halt and said a polite hello. Just like Nitesh, he was busy giving Indian tourists rides along the beach and taking pictures of them on his horse for Instagram.

Things had changed in Agonda. The two years of the pandemic had aged the dogs but it had also brought out a youthful vitality in lots of my Indian friends. At Sampoorna, owner Deepak had lost a huge amount of weight, as had his site manager, Ravi. I barely recognised them – they were half their previous size and they looked so youthful.

"It took a lot of sacrifices!" Ravi said, when I met him in Mandala Café next to Sampoorna. He was beaming with inner light, and couldn't wait to tell me how proud he was of his new wife and baby son. *This is what happiness looks like,* I thought.

Simrose and Kopi Desa were full of Indian tourists and in each, I was one of only a handful of white people. Gone were the boozy Brits, and in their place, a much more respectful crowd. My three-years'-sober self relished the peace of it. In the mornings, the beach was filled with silent people in their pyjamas walking fully clothed into the ocean to start the day, or sitting cross-legged on the sand, staring out at the horizon, a beach dog curled up nearby.

I'd be asked several times if I could 'click a picture' of a couple or a family enjoying the early morning surf and happily agreed. I noticed that I got a 'good morning' from most of the Indians and any white faces studiously ignored me.

The next day, Shubham and I began The Great Return – our programme of visits to our favourite places, starting with Cola Beach. He was clearly determined to make amends for my last trip and began to make space for me in his daytime schedule.

I loved how it felt to have my arms around his waist again as we flew on the Enfield round the winding leafy roads of South Goa. We had a joke about our protruding tummies – I called his Chicken Biryani and he called mine Veg Biryani. If ever I felt scared on the back of the bike, I used the 'full Biryani hold' and wrapped both my arms right round him.

As we bumped over the red rocky ground to the loosely termed 'bike park' above Cola Beach, I smiled and squeezed Shubham round the middle. "Biryani is back," I said, lovingly.

"Dad Bod," Shubham said with a grin, having learned the term from me.

Casa Diya was a new café on the south side of Cola, where we'd stayed in Krishna's hut two years earlier. We ordered masala chai and it came out in two tiny blue and white football-shaped cups. We chinked cups and sipped, staring out at the view between the strands of tiny mirrors dangling from the roof.

"I can't believe I'm here," I said, turning to look at Shubham's profile, his thick eyebrows knitted over his dark eyes in the brightness.

"It is a dream," he replied. "We will wake up soon."

I hope not, I thought.

Just as in Agonda, kayaks had also appeared on the creek at Cola and Shubham managed to speak to someone he vaguely knew, a friend of Ram's, to arrange one for us.

Every Goan we met in the area seemed to be a friend of Ram, Shubham's bar colleague who hailed from nearby Cabo de Rama ('Cab day Ram' when pronounced by locals). Ram was someone who was definitely a dark horse, with his Instagram bio simply stating: *Classified*. No one seemed to know what he did or where he went when he wasn't at Kopi Desa and he liked it that way. I enjoyed teasing him about it: Ram – International Man of Mystery.

We took the kayak upstream, playing 'dodgems' with the

many Indian tourists on the river. We laughed at every bump and splash as we tried to co-ordinate our paddles. It was fun.

I have always been a person who struggles with the idea of fun as larking around, getting wet, getting made fun of, looking stupid. I don't mind watching other people doing it but I really struggle to take part, and I have done since I was a child. I don't laugh at other people's misfortune and I find pranks upsetting. I can't see why you would intentionally make someone else look stupid or even hurt them. I've never enjoyed food or snowball fights or being caught in the rain. To me, they are just messy and annoying, as is being covered in sand on the beach.

To suddenly find myself laughing, soaked to the skin in a kayak, was a release for me. I was playing. Somewhere along the way, I'd forgotten how to do it – in water, on the sand, in the snow – and I realised it had happened after my father died. My mother stopped singing at that time too and when she died, I stopped dancing. In my experience, losing the people who loved you made something inside you die along with them.

Here in Goa, my inner child had been given life again. I'd found ten-year-old Little Lisa during the therapy I'd had in 2018. She had come with me to Goa that Christmas and I'd set her free on its beaches, where she'd skipped away, laughing. She was happy to play on the sand in the bright sunlight in a way I used to in Wales before my father died. It gave me so much joy to see her turn and smile at me before she splashed into the waves.

Whenever Shubham and I went in the sea, I became Little Lisa in his arms. He held me aloft on my back in the waves, like a mermaid with my hair spread out on the water, or let me sit on his hip, my arms circled around his neck, bobbing as each wave rolled past. We'd jump together as a big wave came in and laugh at the dunking we got. He'd emerge like a seal, with glistening black hair and water droplets falling around his face, smiling at me as I spluttered and coughed, making sure my swimwear hadn't been ripped off by the strength of the tide. I'd finally learned to swim a couple of years before but what I liked most of all about being in the sea with Shubham was this return to being a child, someone who could laugh and play and splash around, feeling safe and loved in somebody's arms.

When we were apart, which was a lot of the time in our relationship, Shubham always asked me if I'd had my breakfast, lunch and dinner and made sure I was eating properly. I told him he was like a mother hen; I was so unused to someone asking me if I was eating properly or truly caring about my wellbeing, I didn't know how to respond.

When Shubham gave me the drawings he'd made in quarantine, I'd quietly wondered if I should be pinning them on my fridge door with pride, but I was the infant in this relationship. Almost every day on this trip he would bring me fruit or a smoothie he'd made to put in my little fridge. When he found out I liked samosas with chai and veg pakora we had them almost every day, wrapped up in Hindi newspaper. No man had ever shown such care and his thoughtfulness made my heart (and waistline) swell.

On my 55th birthday, Shubham took me back to Assolna for a fish lunch by the river, just as we had done two years earlier. Embarrassingly, then as now, I found it difficult to navigate a fish with bones in it. Shubham ended up cutting up my fish for me as though I was a child, pulling out all the bones for me. (I still found some though.)

I had 'surprise' chocolate cake three times in total: the

first from Ilu at Mandala at breakfast, the second from
Shubham at Kopi Desa that evening (both occasions
featuring a Happy Birthday singalong from all the staff) and
the third from Simrose the next morning. I revelled in all the
birthday love.

We discovered a new beach near to Agonda – Kakolem –
which had recently been put on the map by Indian Insta-
grammers because it was clearly Paradise Found. Once you'd
bounced your way along the off-road red-dust track, picked
your way down the steep zigzagged steps, crossed the foot of
what would be a waterfall in monsoon but was a small stream
in dry season, you found yourself on the perfect palm-fringed
beach. It had a tiny restaurant, Palm Discoveries, at the back,
with a selection of wooden sunloungers parked between the
angled palms that jutted out over the sand. The waiter,
Dharshan, was a friend of Ram's, obviously.

Shubham positioned a purple umbrella at the foot of my
lounger to protect me from the sun and ordered lime sodas
and vegetable pakoras for after our swim. We bobbed around
in the surf in the safest part of the beach, away from the
rocks, and sat on our loungers to dry off and relax. Sipping
chai an hour or so later, I couldn't remember a time when I'd
felt so happy. Shubham didn't believe me when I told him
how I felt. Surely this couldn't be my happiest day ever?

But it could.

We left the beach as the sun was setting, riding home in
the rose-orange glow of its descent, turning to look at it over
the canopy of the jungle in the valleys and hills below. We
would ride home at this time almost every day of my thirty-
day stay and the little ritual kept a flame alight inside me. I
knew the landmarks of the journey like the back of my hand
and counted them off in my head: the red roof of the Shree

Laxshminarayan temple at Cola; the shop sign on the side of the road that said '*Harsh*'; the bright-yellow bus stop with '*Rise Nation Army*' inexplicably sprayed onto it; the numerous '*Piles Clinic*' posters that made me wonder just how prevalent it was out here; the turning for our favourite Red Crab restaurant and the 'cow corridor' that would fill with the animals in the evening, making Shubham swerve around them as we headed back into Agonda. He told me that the animals were heading for the warm roads, to sleep on during the cool nights. This explained the obstacle course that was nighttime driving in India.

That evening, the traffic jam was caused by Shigmo – the spring festival I'd witnessed two years earlier. I recognised the pleated orange hats of the men, sometimes made from red tinsel, and the slightly military sound of the repetitive drum rhythm that would hit a crescendo with the addition of fire-crackers. The drummers would be visiting all the Hindu households in the village for the next four days until Holi.

I loved this time in Goa for its string of festivities, starting with Shivratri in late February or early March. The special night, '*Maha Shivatri*', means 'the Great Night of Shiva', marking a remembrance of overcoming darkness and igno-rance. On my last visit, I'd missed the ceremony hosted by Ilu in Mandala café so this time I was determined to see what it was all about.

Shiva is the Hindu god that represents the destruction and creation of the universe, his 'cosmic dance' symbolising unity and balance in the world. As the Russian invasion of Ukraine raged far northwest of us, the small group assembled on mats on the café floor witnessed the *puja* – the fire cere-mony representing our connection with the universe. It took place in front of a shrine garlanded in marigolds, representing the power of the sun and the divine light inside all of us.

The celebrant, a young Indian man with a smooth, clear brow, talked of Shiva's 'third eye': his wisdom and ability to see the invisible divine light in all things. He spoke of the power of collective prayer, of honesty, non-injury to others (*ahimsa*), charity and forgiveness. I vowed to learn the Sanskrit words of the *Mahamrityunjaya* Mantra, a verse from the Rig Veda and the most powerful Shiva Mantra. We chanted it 108 times, the numbers 1, 0 and 8 separately signifying 'oneness', 'nothingness' and 'everything' in the ancient scriptures. Together, they represented the ultimate reality of the universe: one, empty and infinite all at the same time. Chanting this mantra 108 times was guaranteed to surround us with Shiva's healing energy, bestowing long life and removing fear.

I continued studying Sudhir's course while in India. I had lost interest in organised religion decades earlier but this philosophy fascinated me. I loved the idea that every living thing is an expression of god – he or she isn't a separate all-powerful deity. God is in all of us, and all of us are god – all we have to do is recognise this divinity in the person or creature in front of us. Not only that, but the core of every living thing is pure – an uninterrupted joy – not an original sin that needs to be atoned for until we're dead. In Hindu philosophy, our only sin is in injuring others, including ourselves. The message of the *Gita* is clear – to be ignorant of our inner godliness is the root of all problems and suffering. And just because living things come in different forms, it doesn't mean they're essentially different.

"Think of a gold bangle," Sudhir said. "The essential thing about it is that it is made from gold, and that gold can be made into a bangle, a ring, and earring, or anything the goldsmith wants to make out of it. But the essential thing itself is gold. All living creatures come in different forms but our essential selves are all made from the same thing: pure consciousness; light, love and joy.

"To be philosophically correct, we should really call a gold bangle, *'bangly gold'*, because the form of the bangle is dependent on it being made from gold, not the other way round."

Bangly gold.

Just before my arrival back in Goa, I'd had a panicked phone call from Shubham. "Everyone knows about us," he'd said. "They've read your book, they've seen the online article!"

I'd written a piece on age-gap relationships for an online newspaper and through the process of Shubham trying to support me on social media by sharing it, his friends and community had discovered and read it. It included pictures of us together at Southampton, which Shubham had approved the use of.

While age-gap relationships between older men and younger women are generally accepted, even if socially side-eyed, a relationship between an older woman and younger man seemed to transgress something much more foundational in society. It was probably the biological role-reversal – an almost-infertile woman with a very fertile man. But I'd been dating younger men for over a decade and knew that there was likely a biological imperative behind it – it felt like it was searching for one last chance to have a baby with the best partner possible. My body didn't know that my brain had decided against that option long ago – it was only doing what came naturally.

Shubham had made me happier than any man my own age and it felt like we existed as a couple in a kind of dream world where social mores didn't matter. When we were flying along Goa's winding roads on the Enfield, nothing else mattered more than me holding on to the laughing man in front of me, taking me for food and making sure I ate all of it, patting my leg if I got scared on the tight bends. Here was a man who made me feel safe, looked after, joyful and desired, but we were both plagued by underlying feelings of uncertainty. We were not allowed to be: it was seen as unnatural. Shubham admitted he was losing sleep over it and I found my joy tainted by the slow drip of 'this isn't forever' sadness.

One afternoon, Shubham came to my room after I'd finished work and we lay facing each other, talking. We tended to avoid talking about the challenges we might face as a couple, but I wanted to know how he felt.

"I don't know what to do," he admitted, wiping a tear from his eye. "I know I want you in my life but ... my community will never accept it. We cannot get married. It's the age-gap, and you are not Hindu. I don't want to upset my father."

We knew that his family knew about us after the newspaper feature went viral here in Goa, but they still hadn't said anything directly to Shubham.

I ran my fingers through his black curly hair, which was getting so long, his friends were referring to him as 'dandelion'. "If you need me to, I will walk away. I will go back to my life in the UK and leave you to find a Goan girl your own age and have a family. It will nearly kill me, but I would do it to see you happy. It was what I was trying to do before, when

I left just before lockdown. I thought it was the universe telling me I couldn't have you."

Shubham rolled on to his back, the black rosary necklace he wore (and often kissed when he took it off) falling onto the pillow. "I don't want to think about the future, about marriage or anything like that. I want to be with you, I want to just live. I would love to come and work in the UK and hike with you in Worthing."

We'd shared a fantasy about Shubham getting a job at a local café or even setting up his own chai and samosa van on the seafront and living with me in my flat. The idea, in our dreams, would be to live in two places, several months of the year in the UK and the dry season in Goa.

"I want the grey weather! I like it. It's too hot here," Shubham said, wiping the sweat from his brow with the sleeve of his *Simpsons* T-shirt.

But somehow I couldn't picture him in the UK, with his dandelion hair, out of his natural habitat of palm trees, Enfield dust tracks and temples filled with colour. At the same time, I couldn't picture myself as one of the ex-pat women who lived in Goa, married to an Indian man, returning to my homeland only sporadically on a visa run. If I was going balance my time between India and UK, I could probably only manage an annual three-month stint in India, and perhaps one of those months in the cooler north, where I'd been planning to visit when the pandemic started.

The idea of a two-centre life had huge appeal. This was a country I loved, but so was back home, hiking in the fresh cool air of spring.

The point of this trip had been to see Shubham while he was on shore leave, to study the *Bhagavad Gita* with Sudhir and to write this book. I was balancing all three and as the final week of my trip approached I focused on Shubham, who seemed more keen to venture off our usual routes and explore more of Goa. It was what I'd wanted all along so I let him lead, as he veered off main roads on to narrow tracks winding through cashew plantations to tiny beaches where he and his friends had come while they were at school. He stopped a cashew farmer to ask him for some fruit for me to try. Pulling off the nut on top of the yellow fruit, Shubham tore a strip and fed it to me. The juice tasted oddly dry, like a green banana. It would be used to make feni, he told me, the local liquor.

A huge banyan tree loomed at us as we turned the bike around on the cashew plantation track and Shubham insisted I pose in front of it, looking up at its long fringed roots, trying to identify the source of the peeping sound I could hear.

"*Tamde lakood*," he said, getting me to turn to the camera. It was my social media name, Redwoods, in Konkani. He knew it would make me smile.

This time we spent Holi doing it right. After a morning spent with his family, Shubham turned up at the Red House at noon, with a bag of the coloured powders, ready to throw over both of us. We decided to spend the day at Kakolem again, which had become our favourite beach, with its steep steps down to a paradise cove and incredible views. Shubham decided to start the festivities as soon as he'd parked the bike above the steps, daubing me with the fuschia pink, yellow, orange and green powders, celebrating the new life and colour of springtime and the blossoming of love.

Shubham had bought two pomfret fish on his way to

meet me, which were immediately handed over to Dharshan
– one fish would be grilled for lunch and one would be made
into a curry for dinner.

After washing off the Holi colours in the ocean, we
settled down onto our loungers with a hot cup of chai,
watching a group of young men carrying supplies over the
rocks to a secluded corner of the beach for a barbecue and
maybe a camp-out.

I looked out over the sparkling ocean and couldn't believe
how different this trip was compared to the ones before it. I'd
been immersed in the yoga world back then, both practising
and teaching, but now I was more likely to find myself medi-
tating on what my future with Shubham would be like, while
sharing a platter of pakora.

Former me would have berated herself for not pushing
herself on to the mat each day. I'd brought two yoga outfits
and hadn't even pulled them out of my case. I knew I
wouldn't. I hadn't stepped on the mat since my book
published, and even though I knew it would be the key to
managing the stress I'd felt, to restoring my peace of mind, I
simply couldn't get myself back on there. Shubham had
mentioned it in almost every call we'd had – *"Why don't
you do some yoga? A bit of meditation?"* – and so had
Miriam. Both of them told me over and over that what I
needed to do was establish some stillness and quiet in my
life.

I thought I was doing that, by spending so much time
alone. I had been on my own almost continuously for
months, only having conversations sporadically with work
clients and people I met on my walks. But Sudhir put me
straight: "Just because you are alone, it does not mean you are
with your self. You can be on your own but be on social

media or watching TV. That is not the same as being with your self."

I thought I had been 'communing' with my self but I hadn't, not really – I'd been filling the void with other things now that I couldn't rely on alcohol to blur reality. Long walks served to energise me and helped me process ideas for my writing, but they were also filled with the internal wrangling of my emotions, which scared me. It was better to be alone, I reasoned, so that they didn't inflict any external damage on anyone.

"Walking is not 'moving meditation'," Sudhir reminded me. "It is mindfulness. Meditation is being, not doing."

I knew that the breathing exercises he'd taught me would reset my body's physical systems and meditation would allow me to untangle my chaotic thoughts and emotions, and slowly shut them down, like tabs closing on an internet browser. But first, I had to roll my mat out and that was the bit that was proving the hardest to do. As Sudhir said, "You can have the knowledge that something is right for you and no doubts about that, but still your habits are strong."

———

On one of our 'glorious return' beach days out, this time to Talpona, I took a walk while Shubham chatted to his cruise-ship friend, Aditya, in Tejas restaurant. I knew they would have a better conversation in Konkani, so I left them to it, to conduct another mindful walk along the wide sands, with barely anyone around me.

As I walked back towards the restaurant in the late-afternoon sun, I watched planes leaving con-trails overhead and noted that things were slowly returning to normal in a post-pandemic world. An elderly white couple emerged onto the sand from the nearby houses where I could see children playing after-school cricket. He was tall and bearded, in a singlet and shorts and a battered cap. She was small and wearing a patterned shift dress to her knees, not unlike the ones Saluzhina and the other women in the Christian community wore (saris were worn by Hindu women).

The man approached me, asking where I was from. Kevin was Australian and his partner, Olly, a Russian. They'd spent lockdown in Talpona with a kind family.

"This place was our saviour," Kevin said, pulling off his cap and smoothing back his thick, greasy, grey hair. He looked rather feral, a Robinson Crusoe of a man. "We love it here and we don't want to leave but I might have to because of my visa. I'm waiting to hear. Now everything is open we get the bus to Margao and buy books from a shop called 'Dog Ears'."

Kevin translated everything I said back to him, about how I was writing a second book and living its content, to Olly in Russian. She smiled at me and nodded, her short grey hair glinting in the sun.

Kevin reminded me of Sven. Here was another man who radiated happiness from every pore. He told me about his extensive travels in his fifties – he'd left work at fifty-seven and never looked back.

"Make the most of the next twenty years, my dear, because in many ways they're the most important," he said, looking at me intently.

"Oh I will," I said, "I will."

As Kevin turned to go, he raised a hand in my direction and clasped the other around Olly's.

"Be joyful!"

On my return to Tejas, Shubham asked me if I'd met some friends.

"No, just another messenger from the universe."

———

The daily exploration of Secret Goa continued, with Shubham's desire to discover the hidden corners of his homeland equalling mine in Wales. His Enfield roared and thumped as it negotiated the ribbon of roads threading through the forested slopes of the Western Ghats. I hadn't even realised, until I looked it up during this trip, that this was a mountain range that runs for 1,000 miles along western India. The Ghats, or the Sayadri mountains, are a UNESCO World Heritage site, and home to an exceptionally high level of biodiversity, among the world's top eight. They have a huge influence on the monsoon weather pattern and are older than the Himalayas. In staying on the coast, I'd missed this incredible hinterland, filled with life, human and animal, and now was the time to correct that.

We rode to Cotigao Wildlife Sanctuary, the nearest nature reserve, taking in Chapoli Dam, one of our previous haunts, on the way. It served the Canacona district, including Palolem and Agonda, with its drinking water, and had views of the mountain range. I remembered wearing what could only be described as a *Great Escape* bike helmet on my previous visit and Shubham had taken some awkward pictures of me by the water. My skin was exceptionally pale and I was stiff with fright after being on the bike. What a different picture that was now, with a veil of golden freckles across my face, arms and legs, and no stiffness at all. I'd relaxed on the bike, finally.

"I can tell when you're just holding me with love and not scared," Shubham said. "You squeeze my chicken biryani."

It was true. As we coursed around the surprisingly freshly tarmacked roads, I squeezed him affectionately around his middle and smiled. He was showing me his homeland and it was everything.

"You should see this place in monsoon!" he cried, pointing at some rolling fields in the foothills of the ghats. An evening mist was already beginning to settle and I wondered how much more beautiful it could get.

It was the time of day when the golden-furred langur monkeys began their evening commute among the trees. I'd watched them use the roofs of Sampoorna as staging posts on the hill of the yoga school. They never stopped to pinch our banana and biscuit snacks – I'm still puzzled as to why not.

It was also the time of day for *puja* – I could hear the bells ringing as people walked, cycled and scooted towards local temples. At roadside shrines, incense puffed into the air and golden vessels containing small fires were offered before deities garlanded in marigolds. It seemed that all around there was yellow.

The roads were bordered with the blossom of the tall trees that arched over them, creating golden holloways I wish we could have ridden through forever. I got off the bike and walked among them, wondering what the trees were called.

"Shiva trees," Shubham said, straddling the bike as he clicked pictures of me.

Shiva – the universal consciousness, the totality. *Ishvara*. The god in all of us and in every living thing. At that very moment I could hear it – the universal *Om*, the sound of the totality – in the hum of life all around us.

A small girl gazed at us shyly from a house behind a

cluster of mango trees heavy with green fruit. She had a T-shirt with '*Cute Girl*' written on it. Shubham spoke to her in Konkani, encouraging her to join me for a photo but she was too shy to. I knew that one day she would have the confidence have her picture taken with a stranger.

As I walked back towards Shubham my mind showed me an image of myself at the girl's age, perhaps ten years old, the age I'd been when my father had died. Here I was at fifty-five, about to get on the back of a motorbike with my Goan boyfriend of twenty-seven. I could never ever have predicted this moment, and I hoped the 'cute girl' had the same surprises in store for her, but without the pain of losing her parents so early.

I approached the bike. "Where next?"

"I don't know, babe," he said. "We'll just flow like water. Oh I forgot! I have something for you," he cried, turning and opening a tiny compartment in the side of the bike and holding a brown paper bag out towards me.

For a moment, I thought it was yet more pakora, but I slid my hand into the bag and pulled out two golden bangles, studded with shining diamond-like stones that shone in the evening sun.

"Bangly gold," he said, smiling, pushing them one by one onto my wrist.

WORTHING, WEST SUSSEX
APRIL-MAY 2022

ONE OF THE NEW PLACES SHUBHAM HAD TAKEN ME TO in Goa was a house-cum-shop in the countryside near Chaudi that was filled with things I wanted to buy. From Himalayan blankets and hemp bags, to mirrored beads and embroidered notebooks, this place had it all. The stock was piled high across three rooms of a huge bright-green Portuguese villa nestling among the trees. Children played outside near a shrine to Shiva and a huge sleeping dog lay across the entrance to the main room. I stepped over him to get through.

Now, I placed the shiny, colourful things I'd bought around my tiny flat in Worthing and once again, the place filled with Goan warmth, colour and love.

Just before I left Goa, worried friends messaged me about my emotional state, knowing what it had been like for me leaving Goa pre-pandemic. Every single time it had felt like I was being ripped apart but something changed this time. I was much much calmer. On those previous occasions, I'd been unable to handle the idea of never seeing the place, people or animals ever again and a torrent of emotion had burst out of me at the very idea. Shubham was at the apex of that torrent, sitting atop the wave as it crested each time I was due to leave. He couldn't bear seeing me cry and kept asking me to stop, but I couldn't. Except this time, I did.

This time I knew for sure that I was definitely going to see him, and Agonda, again. There was no doubt, no pandemic to hold me back. If anything, I was even more sure of my love for Shubham. This trip had, underneath it all, been a bit of a make-or-break scenario for me. I was still wondering if my feelings for Shubham could exist in a real world beyond a fantasy location, and for the first time, I had allowed myself to think of a possible future with him. We had actually talked about it. I hadn't dared to do that up until this point, too worried about what people might think and too afraid of making a fool of myself. There had been no backlash from the online article about us. No one had said anything to Shubham about it, other than his friends. I was more in love than ever. So was he.

Friends asked me how I felt, if I was bereft to be so far away from him, but the truth was I still felt connected to Shubham. We were two sparks of energy, of pure consciousness, that just happened to be located in two bodies, on two different continents, in two different age groups and two different societies. Even when we were apart, we felt this connection and it left neither of us bereft, because we were always there for each other.

Miriam called this a 'twin flame' scenario, when two souls are divinely connected, aware of each other's presence at all times, even when not together. When it came to Shubham and me, our 'flames' flickered for each other wherever we were. It didn't matter to us that we were so far apart for so long and with a slim-to-zero chance of being accepted by society, because they were superficial restrictions when it came to the universal picture. We saw each other everywhere – I saw Shubham in the sparkling light on the sea every morning and the dandelions lining the coastal path. They made me smile as their seed clocks gave way to their bright yellow flowers. Sadly, Shubham's hair had been cut for his next cruise – so it would be a while before he became 'dandelion' again.

Yellow flowers were everywhere that spring. On my weekend hikes on the South Downs I was walking alone among daffodils, dandelions, buttercups and daisies and fields full of rapeseed flowers either side of the path. So much yellow. So much of my darling waving at me in the breeze. He'd call me from the ship while I was hiking, pulling off his cap to reveal shorn hair. We joked about him looking like a young Indian Elvis. I'd show him where I was walking on my phone camera and he would say, "I wish I was there."

"You are," I'd say. *You are.*

I'd continued with Sudhir's course back in England and I loved the concept that we exist in pure consciousness before the birth of our bodies and continue to exist after death. *"The body is simply a shell that houses this consciousness,"* Sudhir said.

As someone who'd dealt with a lot of death in her life the concept of this infinite consciousness – which I now thought of as 'yellow', from sparks of sunlight to the smallest flower – had helped me think about grief in a different way. I had always thought of my parents as still being around me, even though they were not physically there – I'd even felt them from time to time, usually in the wind. And now I knew that they were.

I'd clearly felt my mother's presence with me on the Helvellyn range in the Lake District on a solo hike the previous year. I can't explain it – I suddenly felt her there, just her, on her own. It was just a very strong feeling, just like the one I'd had in Morfa Bychan in North Wales before I published my first book. I could feel that she was happy and I wasn't scared by her presence.

I'd been scared of seeing the ghost of my father when I was a little girl, not realising that he would return as an unseen presence much later. He came to me once before I published *Cheat Play Live*, near my favourite area of my morning walk: the World War Two pillbox in Ferring. It was a brief encounter. Having fought in that war himself, maybe he thought it was a good idea to meet me there. His was a calming, reassuring energy; there was something grounding about it. It came at a time when I was concerned about the backlash against my book.

Sudhir said that there was a reason why the *Bhagavad Gita* deals with the sorrow of one man, Arjuna. "Sorrow is a fundamental human experience that makes us stop and ask ourselves the deeper questions about our lives," he said. "It reminds us that we have much to be grateful for and how much we take for granted. Sorrow is an opportunity to learn, for all of us."

Grief was just one aspect of sorrow – we could feel sorrowful over the loss of family, a friendship, the failure of a relationship or even the loss of status in an industry. I had felt sorrow over all those things and the mistake I'd often made was to think I was alone.

One of the first things I did when I got back from Goa was to see a doctor. I'd experienced a set of symptoms there that told me something was wrong. I'd felt a little nauseous every day, I felt bloated and full very quickly after eating and I was experiencing a dull ache in the left side of my abdomen after sex. It passed quickly, but I was worried enough about all of this to get a pregnancy test while I was out there. I knew my chances were below 1% at fifty-five, but I knew I'd be incredibly anxious if I didn't check.

Shubham offered to buy the tests and brought two, wrapped in newspaper, to my room. They looked like the lateral flow tests from back home. I asked him what he would do if it was positive and he said, "I'd pack a bag, leave Goa and come and look after you."

Part of me knew I wouldn't be able to go through with a pregnancy (my instinct to stay childfree has always been strong) but part of me also painted a picture of a child that looked like me and Shubham, playing in the Goan sunshine. That would have to wait until we were reincarnated in another life. It wasn't going to happen in this one and I felt unexpectedly sad about it. The tests, taken days apart, were negative.

I googled my symptoms and saw that they were in line with ovarian cancer so decided to see a doctor as soon as possible on my return. I'd also had a 'period' two weeks before the trip and at the end of the trip – I dismissed them because the HRT nurse had told me to expect some 'surprise' bleeding, but I threw them into my list of symptoms when I called her.

"You shouldn't be bleeding at all, Lisa," she said, suddenly serious.

"But you told me to expect the Biblical floods from time to time?"

"That's in the first few months. You've been on HRT for a year now. There should be no bleeding."

She immediately booked me a blood test and and emergency appointment with the doctor, who examined me and couldn't find anything immediately wrong. But she promptly booked me an ultrasound scan and made me do another pregnancy test: negative again.

Shubham and I laughed nervously on the phone about it as I walked home. He told me I would be fine, as he always did. "Don't worry about anything. Don't stress. Flow like water."

I was impressed by the speed of it all, until I realised that this also meant that they thought I could have cancer. At least the blood test came back normal.

The day of the scan came around and I joked as best I could with the radiologist and her assistant as they balanced my bottom on a foam wedge and prepared the scanner, which would inserted inside me. I'd had to make sure my bladder was 'uncomfortably full', which was fairly easy for someone my age, and when I asked why, the radiologist said that they look through it to view the reproductive organs. It has to be distended for them to see everything clearly.

My scan showed 'pelvic congestion', a fairly common condition that I'd never heard of, particularly as it mainly affects women with a few children under their belts.

"It's like varicose veins but on the left side of your womb," the radiologist said. "Nothing sinister."

I started googling as soon as I left the hospital, relieved that no weird tumour of mass had shown itself on the scan. It made sense because that's where I could feel the dull ache from time to time.

As a treat, and as a small celebration, I bought myself a raspberry tart in a café in Shoreham-by-Sea and sat at the bar in the window with my legs dangling off a tall stool, watching the world go by. I wondered how many of the women of my age had had some sort of reproductive issue during their lifetimes. Probably all of them.

As I got home my phone started ringing.

"Hello, it's your doctor."

"Oh, that was quick! I've only just got back. I know about the pelvic congestion," I said brightly.

"There's something else I'm concerned about," she said, curtly interrupting me. "Your womb lining is thicker than it should be and that's a symptom of uterine cancer. I'd like to refer you to a consultant within two weeks for a biopsy."

I know that like me, friends who've lost parents, or anyone dear to them, are able to understand and relate like no other group of people can. If you're 'lucky', this happens later in life, but for some, like me, it happens when you're a child. When I had therapy back in 2018, I dismissed the effect that it had had on my life but my therapist had insisted on talking about it. It'd had such a marked effect, it was almost too big to see.

It's said that if you make it through your fifties – the sniper years – alive, you might live for very long time, but my dad died at fifty-eight from bowel cancer. Every now and again, I'd have a dark night of the soul and wake up worrying that I'd die like him, or risk living another twenty years with slowly encroaching dementia, as my mother had. Surely one or the other would get me. My research told me that a history of bowel cancer could be a risk factor for uterine cancer – was this the thing that would get me in the end? I thought I'd got home and dry with no problematic smear tests – cervical cancer being a more significant problem in women under fifty. How was I to know that there would be a whole new uterine cancer threat to deal with in my fifties? It seemed like no one ever talked about it.

I worried that the thing that had made this all happen was the HRT – perhaps it wasn't all it was made out to be and I was paying the price. Perhaps the Covid vaccine had messed around with my menstruation, as it had for many women around the world. I had so many questions, but I was told to wait until I saw the consultant. I looked up my record online and clicked on 'Consultations'. It said, "referral due to suspected gynaecological cancer." I immediately made my will online.

I'd texted a few friends to let them know what was happening. None of them had heard of pelvic congestion but some had mothers who'd had uterine cancer issues them-selves. They reassured me and told me to keep them posted. I told them I felt surprisingly ok about it and I meant it – researching all the information on it all reassured me that my doctor was making extremely sensible checks given the presenting symptoms. I had to be patient while what needed to be done was done.

But my anxiety levels diverted themselves to other areas instead, filling another huge bag of worries. There is no doubt that HRT had got me to the stage where my emotions were more manageable, but it wasn't enough to contain them. I was having another round of work-related emotional flare-

ups which resulted in tears of frustration (upsetting Shubham, who witnessed them because he was the only person I
was confiding in) and a crisis of confidence.

I'd opted out of corporate life and at times it felt like I'd
made a huge mistake, because now I felt I was a nobody,
sitting at my kitchen table writing and self-publishing books
that no one wanted to read and looking and sounding useless
in Zoom meetings with clients. I knew this was my ego
speaking, but I started tuning into its insidious voice: "*You
know you're not good enough, don't you? You know that no
one likes you, don't you? They've found out what you're really
like. You're a nightmare to work with or be friends with. Why
would anyone bother? Best if you stay away from everyone.*"

On my solo hikes, I was still going over and over the
events of the previous year, picking over the debris of my
failed friendships, relationships and beginning to turn the
spotlight on myself. I was the common denominator in all
this – and as I pounded through the miles of chalk paths on
the South Downs, I concluded that I must be a terrible,
deeply flawed person who couldn't hold on to a friendship, a
relationship or a job. I wanted to hide until it was all over.

Before therapy and yoga had helped me take it down, I'd
built a fortress around myself after my dad died and kept it
there for decades, adding to it stone by stone until no one
could see the real me – Little Lisa – hiding inside. Little Lisa
had finally broken through the walls in Goa but now she was
furiously building them back up again. By exposing my dark
horses in my first book I'd made myself vulnerable again. So I
started rebuilding the fortress, trying to protect myself from
unseen enemies. But when I looked around, the only enemy
in sight was me.

I told myself that I loved being alone, scuttling out for

my walk every day like a crab leaving its shell and retreating back to my desk, avoiding any major encounters with anyone. I found it easier to be on my own than deal with foulweather friendships or fake relationships. It was simpler just to hide from everyone. I was aware enough to know that I was distancing myself from people who mirrored aspects of myself back at me. It was my deepest fear that I was the one who was jealous, competitive and judgemental. I railed so hard against these things that it told a story I wasn't even willing to tell myself. My tiny flat was my sanctuary. I could hide from any potential hurt and at the same time, I could prevent myself from hurting other people.

But however much I tried, I couldn't escape myself. I found it impossible to sit on my yoga mat and truly face myself so the only peace of mind I found was in my bed and I slept every night like a baby. Every day I moved from my bed to my walk to my work and back to bed again and the amount of time I was spending alone in my flat was increasing. Was I becoming a hermit like my mother? Would I retreat, retreat and retreat some more until I was barely a shadow?

The appointment for my biopsy came around one Saturday morning in May. I'd researched pelvic congestion and uterine cancer thoroughly and actually found the results encouraging. There was a very slim 3% chance that I'd develop uterine cancer at my age, and I received a reassuring letter from the hospital that said, '*The majority of patients seen in our clinics do not have cancer. The purpose of our clinic is to try and identify what is causing your symptoms as quickly as possible so that we can try and resolve them for you.'*

My main concern was that the HRT was causing my issues – I could see that for both conditions, a high level of oestrogen was responsible, but there again, the progesterone part of my patch, Norethisterone, also caused post-menopausal bleeding.

As I'd done when I stopped drinking, I joined an online forum where I could anonymously ask questions. The women on there, or should I say the people with uteruses on there, reassured me that my patch was delivering a very low amount of oestrogen and an amount of progesterone that would offset any imbalance. The patch was probably not causing the issue.

It was clear that they knew their stuff because the gynae-cological consultant said the same thing. My patches were low delivery – in fact, he thought the problem might be *not enough* oestrogen. When I reported my high levels of anxi-ety, he said it was a classic sign. I'd just come out of a week where I'd cried every day at something that didn't warrant it.

The day before the biopsy I'd spent two hours crying about being the world's worst person. I thought about all the times I'd been critical or lashed out at someone and suddenly saw myself as the ultimate Mean Girl. Yes, I'd done and said some mean things, but I was being horribly unfair to myself. I was also wallowing, and when I saw my mascara-streaked face in the mirror, I knew I was under hormonal control. But, as with PMS, the feelings were incredibly real, just hugely magnified.

I asked the consultant about whether or not a blood test could assess my levels of oestrogen, but he said that they were so prone to change on a daily basis, that they wouldn't be conclusive enough. Most of the diagnosis done in clinics went off a patient's symptoms, he said, from bleeding to joint pain, hot flushes and the rest. I also asked him if it was annoying to have someone come in who'd done a load of research and wanted answers on things like this. "No," he said, "it actually helps because we can move the conversation much further along."

The consultant extracted a small amount of tissue from my womb lining in a process that gave me painful stomach cramps while it was happening – so much so that I started chanting mantras out loud and practising yogic breathing. I had my hands pressed together in prayer position over my heart. It was like a painful smear test, but it was over relatively quickly. He said I'd have the results in three weeks – he was checking to make sure that the cells in the lining of my womb were not cancerous or pre-cancerous.

I cried after the biopsy – I blamed a lack of oestrogen of course – but it was really because I felt very alone. I had very supportive friends waiting for news on WhatsApp but Shubham was out at sea. I desperately wanted someone, for once, to be by my side and hold my hand and say that everything was going to be ok. I had a strong sense that it would be, but my family history was preying on my mind, and making me wonder if my time was up. Word had come through to me of an ex-colleague who died from a particularly virulent form of bowel cancer. She was the same age as me.

The sniper years.

———

Menopause was now being talked about everywhere, led by TV presenter Davina McCall's high-profile investigations.

Many women were sharing their stories, not only in my anonymous forum, but around the world on social media. We were discovering we weren't alone.

I remembered a member of my team going through it, unable to come into work because she couldn't stop crying. She told me she'd been prescribed anti-depressants by her doctor. Back then, only four years earlier, no one had even said the word 'menopause'. I found myself whispering the problem to HR and describing it in code to my male boss who finally understood. It was handled sympathetically by the HR department, but there were looks passing among the management team that said, '*Oh dear, she's going through 'the change'.*'

There was a sense that once these words were spoken out loud, our shelf lives in the workplace – and in the world at large – were over. In the corporate world, women going through these issues would be expected to slide away quietly into the background, and they often did, pushed gently to the blurry sidelines by other, younger, more power-hungry women and men.

Hearing other women's stories made me think about how much of my recent working life had been hormonally driven. In the last few years, working in toxic office environments, I had been unable to handle the pressure, which often led to misguided emotional outbursts. Now I was sure that my hormones were responsible for them, at least to some extent. My perimenopause had probably started around five years earlier – probably around the time my joint pain started in my shoulders. How much better might I have been able to cope with stress if I'd had HRT back then?

I thought about my mother, who'd endured her own menopause in silence, living with her pubescent daughter who was at the other end of the hormonal spectrum, mirroring her yo-yo-ing emotions and moods. My mother's generation had been scared off HRT by alleged cancer risks. It did appear that there was a slight link between some cancers – ovarian and uterine – with HRT but other factors, such as weight, family history and lifestyle choices came into play in a much more significant way. Ironically, I also knew I was at a higher risk of both because I'd never had children. But I was determined to tell every woman I knew about my symptoms and tell them to get checked out if they had the same. We shouldn't all have to suffer the same fate in silence.

I slowly worked through the modules of Sudhir's course while waiting to hear about my results. I realised that the emotional torrents I was experiencing – of grief, anger, sadness and anxiety – were not just governed by phases of the moon or by my menopausal hormone levels; they were also governed by me, and I had the power to channel them in any way I wanted to.

In the *Gita*, Arjuna suffers from an 'emotional hijack' on the morning before a battle, panicking about what to do. Krishna, his teacher, advocates emotional awareness, control and balance.

"If you know that your true self is pure bliss," Sudhir explained, "then emotions are just a distortion of that, like putting a filter on your selfie. You can take the filter off and be your true self. Think of it also like a mirror with marks on it – you can wipe the mirror clean."

There were Six Enemies of Peace, he went on: emotions that rob us of our inner joy. I'd been using similar words ever since I'd published my book, telling friends that I'd felt robbed of my peace of mind. Here were the same words, used in a 5,000-year-old text.

The first three enemies were the three gateways to hell Sudhir had already told me about: intense craving (*kaama*), greed (*lobha*) and anger (*krodha*). I related hard with my corporate career and my alcohol addiction and I'd kicked both of those, but a sugar addiction (very common in sobriety) and menopausal anger were still rearing their heads from time to time.

Next came delusion (*moha*), a denial or refusal to acknowledge that the thing you want is bad for you, then arrogance (*mada*), thinking you are better than someone else because you have what they want. And finally, *matsarya* – a beautiful name for such an ugly enemy – jealousy. I had witnessed all of these things in myself and other people.

Now I had a list of Six Enemies to vanquish on my own personal battlefield. Somehow naming them and writing them down – as has always been the case with me – made them something I'd be able to deal with. I would use them as a checklist for everything I did from that moment on. They wouldn't ever completely go away, Sudhir said, because all (unenlightened) humans are prone to them, but I could learn to manage and control them. He'd once told me that he had learned to conquer jealousy. Sudhir was a former monk but he'd also been a man with a career just like mine, managing his own emotions in the battlefield of corporate life.

Learning about the Six Enemies unblocked something inside me. For the first time in months, I rolled my thick, black rubber Sampoorna mat out on the floor next to my desk and found my yoga blocks. I modified everything on the mat to my less-than-flexible body as usual. I would practice '*ahimsa*' and be kind to myself – I knew my body would have stiffened up again, after all the sitting at my desk and walking.

I was surprised to find that it hadn't. In fact, something felt easier about it. Perhaps because my expectation of myself had shifted and I felt more grateful for the things that my body *could* do, using the blocks and straps to help it.

I added on a breath practice and a meditation called the *Pancha Kosha*, which worked through five 'layers': from the outside world, through the physical body, the breath and the mind to the shining, untarnished gem of the blissful self inside. It was a process that forced me to witness my thoughts, emotions and beliefs, all of which were not my true self. These things were just filters, programmed into me by lived experience, waiting to be witnessed, acknowledged and cleared away, like marks on a mirror.

The effect of my Six Enemies list was not only felt on the mat. I started cooking healthier meals for myself, having suddenly got the urge to start. I'd always thought that cooking for myself was a waste of time and been in denial (*moha!*) about the ill effects my diet of largely processed food was having on me for years. I'd never been able to understand people who told me they found cooking therapeutic, but now I began to look forward to the moment when I would select a recipe and start chopping vegetables in my tiny kitchen while listening to an audiobook. I realised what they'd been talking about all this time.

I tried to work out why I'd been so reliant on processed food, particularly since my marriage had ended over a decade ago. Back then, I'd been on an almost constant low-carb diet so was often creating healthier meals by default – fish and veg mainly – throwing a box of oven chips into the microwave for my more carb-needy husband. But after I left him, I found I couldn't be bothered cooking, especially as there was a convenient supermarket underneath my flat in Kensal Rise where I could buy food that simply needed heating up. Often, I'd look in my huge fridge-freezer and see nothing but prosecco, a block of cheese and ready meals.

Then I remembered that my mother had slowly given up on eating healthy food when I was a teenager. She hated the confines of the kitchen. While my dad had been alive, she reluctantly made dinners in her pressure cooker, which steamed away while the shipping forecast was read out on the radio. But after he died, she began to rely on canned and potted products: fish, soups, yoghurts topped off with a night-time cereal bowl (because her diet left her hungry) and copious biscuits. I'd subconsciously picked up on her routine.

Once I started cooking for myself, trying out simple Indian recipes at first, I realised that fresher food meant a fresher me. I felt warm and well when I made myself nutritious meals, and I liked the idea of helping my body fight whatever was going on inside it.

How had I got to fifty-five without knowing how good this was for me? Like my mum, I had completely stopped caring about myself; but unlike her, I had the opportunity to change the programme. I might be in my sniper years, but I would do my best to avoid the gunfire.

One evening after yoga, I received a video call from Shubham. I told him how happy I was to be back on the mat and garbled what I'd learned about the Six Enemies from the *Bhagavad Gita*.

"You know more than me!" he cried.

But I knew that the values in the story were embedded in him from birth – I could see it in the way he handled his emotions and acted selflessly – except for when his 'volcano' temper got the better of him. It was a dark horse that stalked him sometimes. We were more similar than we realised – in certain situations he'd bottle all his negative emotions up inside until they blew up and out over everyone around.

"Have you had your dinner?" he asked, as he did every time he called. He'd been horrified at some of the processed food I ate.

"Yes! I made it myself," I answered proudly. "Sweet potato and lentil dhansak."

"You are almost Goan!" he said laughing.

He told me he'd said '*gishgogerysh*' to a Welsh couple who'd promptly given him a gift of a pen with Caernarfon Castle on it. I imagined their shock as he suddenly said the Welsh words. He'd told them about me and my book, forever my personal marketing and PR person.

"The lady has the shiny patch! Just like yours!"

"What?!"

"The one on your heep!"

My HRT patch? How on earth had he even spotted it on another woman?! I daren't ask.

"She asked me if I knew what it was…" he said, grinning.

"Oh my god, she didn't!! What did you say?!"

"It's Stroppy Cow! Just like my girlfriend!"

Running away is something I do when times get tough. I ran away from Wales as a young woman, to get away from my depressing existence. I'd literally started running for exercise in my thirties to get away from my unhappy marital home, then I ran away from my husband to explore what I thought might be greener pastures. More recently, I'd run away from corporate life because I couldn't stand the pressure and and now, with my health hanging in the balance, I was considering running once again.

When I returned from Goa, I had an urge to start again somewhere else. I longed for the life of a nomad where you didn't stay in the same place for too long, nor became too attached to other people there, which I tended to do. I had an all-or-nothing approach to friendships and relationships that was highly intense. I had a tendency to break them because I shared too much and expected too much back; I couldn't seem to have them in moderation – a bit like my previous relationship with alcohol. Why have one glass when you can have the bottle?

I reread one of my favourite novels, *Chocolat* by Joanne Harris, and envied the life of the protagonist, Vianne, who constantly moves around the world with her young daughter, never putting down roots. Vianne reminded me of myself, travelling to India with Little Lisa.

A fellow yogi friend, Gail – whom I nicknamed Guru Gail – reminded me that I could be that nomad. I had no family responsibilities to tie me here – not even a pet – my stuff was still (mostly) in storage and I could work anywhere in the world, now it was opening up again. Why not? What was I waiting for?

"It's not running away," she said, in one of our many WhatsApp chats where I expressed my concerns. *"It's choosing freedom."*

Freedom. All I needed was wifi and my Macbook. I knew

I could do it, and it would be exciting. I'd be living the dream again! But I'd had a taste of that and I knew that it was far from dreamlike. Wherever I went in the world, my dark horses still galloped round me, because I was the one they were tethered to. And I would meet people who would mirror them back to me, who would make me want to run from the sound of their hooves again.

But still, I dreamt of escaping to Wales and living in a tiny home there. I'd loved my stay in Louise and Eric's shepherd's hut and the Hobbit house of the couple who'd offered me tea in Llanddona. I longed to just plant myself near the beach in a tiny trailer, get all of my stuff out of storage and then get rid of most of it. Since extracting a small amount of it to ride out the pandemic in Worthing, I hadn't needed anything.

I wondered why I was holding on to boxes and boxes of books, photo albums, memorabilia, wedding tableware and my mum's old tea sets. I know what Sudhir would've said – allowing yourself to become too attached to physical things only brought suffering. It was hardly suffering, but the £100 I was paying for storage every month on top of my rent wasn't exactly bringing me joy either. Every now and again I'd think of my carefully collected Royal Ballet programmes sitting in a plastic tub in a pod in Guildford and think: *why?*

The taxi driver who'd taken me to Heathrow for my trip to Goa told me that he and his wife were moving out of their big family home into a trailer. "Yeah, me and the wife don't need all that space anymore. We can use the money to support our sons' families and live happily near the sea. All we need to do is leave it empty for two weeks a year, which is easy – we'll just go on holiday!"

For me, the trailer idea had been a pipe dream but here was someone who was actually doing it.

"You should see it – it comes with all mod cons! Bluetooth and a wet room."

I'd seen these things on Instagram, where I obsessed over the tiny-home phenomenon. I clearly wasn't the only one who desired to live a simpler, less-cluttered life. I dreamed of having a tiny home both in Wales and in Goa, and shuttling between the two.

I told Shubham about the conversation and he was all for it. "That's what I want," he said. "I don't need anything. I don't need stuff. I just want a space to live and be happy. Maybe a garden to grow things."

Shubham and I also discussed the plan of him coming to live with me for part of the year in the UK. But could this really happen? Was I still being ridiculous, thinking that I could actually set up any sort of life with a twenty-eight-year-old Indian man? For one thing, I wasn't even sure if I'd be around to see it through.

I confided in my therapist friend, Helen, who'd always been supportive of my relationship with Shubham and of my book. She was a fellow Indiaphile and I was round at her flat in St Leonard's sipping her homemade chai on her sunny balcony. She'd just got back from Sri Lanka.

"What's the worst that will happen? You'll live some life," she said matter-of-factly. "It might be three weeks, three months, three years or thirty years. Any of those options will be worth it."

I laughed as she said it but she was so beautifully right.

Live some life.

Why was I ladling so many anxieties over it all, yet again? I'd already batted away so many of society's issues with how I'd chosen to live, but there seemed to be another layer, and it was programmed deep inside myself. I was the one putting up the barriers, not 'society'. I was beginning to learn that I was the sole agent of my life, and I was the one limiting my horizons, however much I blamed a faceless 'society' for it. All this time I had thought of myself as truly free, throwing the shackles off what was expected of a forty- and fiftysomething woman, when all along, I was still wearing the shackles and holding my own key.

Sudhir taught me that freedom can be found in the realisation that I am connected to the world and every living thing in it by the divine light of pure consciousness. "Think of a wave," he said. "The wave may look around at other waves and think, *Hey, I'm a wave!* but that thought restricts the wave and limits its potential to only being a wave. In essence, the wave is water. The wave is only truly free when it identifies as water."

I am not a wave, I am water.
Flow like water.

There is a word in Welsh – *hiraeth* – that doesn't have a direct English translation. It has been described as a deep longing for home – my dad described it to me as '*a longing for the hills*'. But it has a deeper meaning; it is a longing to be where your spirit lives, a yearning to return to a place that has now gone, like a childhood home. I knew where my spirit lived – on a beach in Agonda and on a windswept peninsula in Wales. And the souls of my parents and my ten-year-old self followed me to those places, waiting for me to choose a place to rest, to call my own.

One day in May, in a moment of typical procrastination at my desk, I idly search flats to rent in North Wales. One flat popped up – it was in a new-build near a beach I loved, and available for rent. *What am I waiting for?* I thought.

I looked outside at my garden as a hedgesparrow and a pigeon picked their way around the ground underneath the birdfeeder, picking up scraps. Worthing and this flat had been a good home to me during lockdown and I'd found real joy here, in friendships and my walks on the seafront and on the Downs; even during lockdown in the tiny confines of my rooms and garden. I knew it would always be special to me, but it wasn't my forever home.

Shubham, determined to see me happy and smiling, encouraged me to find that home and approved of the Welsh flat.

"But what about all my stuff?" my oestrogen-deprived brain whined. "What about not having a car? I haven't driven for years!"

"Babe, just flow like water. You will be happy there, I know it. All I want is for you to be happy. My smiling Lisann."

I took a risk, putting an offer on the flat without the results of my biopsy coming through. The universe was begging me to go back to my homeland and the *hiraeth* was strong. I cried – probably the low oestrogen again.

The flat wouldn't be my forever home, but it would be a home in the right place, by a windswept beach where I could see the mountains of Snowdonia National Park in the distance. I worked out that my hometown would be just over an hour away, as were Aberdaron and Snowdon. If I bought myself a car, I could drive to all of them at weekends, even weekdays, if I fancied it. I dreamt of having a little dog – a Jack Russell – in the car with me, ready to accompany me on adventures. A new life back in my homeland was beckoning. My parents were waiting and Little Lisa wanted to run free there. I could live out my days there, however many I was destined to have.

As I'd done in my London flat three years before, I planned to slowly rid myself of the burden of things that I'd collected around myself during lockdown: a slow accretion of papers, books, excess fittings from flat-packed furniture and electrical fittings leftover from appliance purchases that I thought I 'might need' one day. Once again, I would experience the relief of ridding myself of them, wondering why I was so wired to keep things. Perhaps it was an ancient element of our DNA, collecting things that might come in useful as we hunted and gathered. Not having 'stuff' to plant down in a space leaves us feeling without roots and without a home, and yet I'd been at my happiest with barely anything.

In my next move I wanted to see if I could slowly get rid of everything I had in storage, apart from my mum and dad's memorabilia and heirlooms. I wanted to give everything away and live simply near a beach, especially if I didn't have much time left. I wanted to begin the task of slowly getting rid of everything until I'd boiled my life down to essentials 'plus'; the 'plus' being some of my favourite books, my Indian things, and my mother's tableware.

I wondered if a café in Wales would offer to stock my books and if I could make a whole new set of friends, avoiding scaring them away with the intensity of my emotions and sharing too much of myself at the same time.

That seemed to be where my problem lay – people didn't always know how to handle my dark horses because I didn't have them under control myself.

And then, a phone call.

"Miss Edwards? I have the results of your biopsy. I'm pleased to confirm that it has shown no abnormality. It's clear."

EPILOGUE

A SECOND PHONE CALL WAS FROM THE PROPERTY AGENT in Wales who confirmed that the flat I'd put an offer on was now for sale. It was not meant to be. I knew that my destiny was to end up back in Wales, but not yet. I'd rushed at it because I'd been fleeing from my health problems, but it would happen. *In time, my love, in time.*

I desperately wanted to tell Shubham that my biopsy results had come in and that they were negative, but he had gone silent, even though I could see his ship plodding around the Mediterranean on my ship-tracker app. His SIM card had clearly run out, as it did from time to time.

I smiled when I thought about the timing of his silence – the same thing had happened when I needed to focus on finishing *Cheat Play Live* and now it was happening with its sequel, this book. The universe was up to its old tricks again.

The news of my all-clear made me renew a vow to myself to live some life. I would stay connected with the world, not only through my breath and meditation practice but as a human engaging with other humans in the real world, not just on social media. I would Be More Bram and find more freedom and happiness in the service of others – I had tangible evidence that this was a Karma Yoga strategy that worked for me. I wanted to help other people tell their stories and knew I had the skills to offer. I would publish this book to tell other women that their symptoms had a name – and a potential solution. It would be my second child in the world and I would make sure it had the very best start in life.

I felt ready to face the world again, with a renewed sense of who I was, both physically and emotionally. I had shed another layer that I no longer needed, like a lizard in the sun. I would crawl out and be the person I was underneath all the life programming I'd experienced, fresh and new, eating healthily, managing my hormones with the right HRT, walking and taking good care of myself. I knew that if I was going to be kinder to others, it would start with being kinder to my fifty-five-year-old self. For now, my dark horses were stabled and resting.

The following weekend I took myself high onto the Downs and gazed over the buttercup-filled fields on either side of the chalk path. Everywhere was yellow, the space between spring and summer; everywhere was hope and renewal. I thought of Shubham and felt him by my side.

I was loitering by a gate crowded by large cows on one side, afraid to walk through in case I'd get trampled. I smiled as I recalled Sudhir trying to say the word 'cow' in a Western way – to rhyme with 'now' rather than 'know'.

While I was considering my options, a woman my age with silver hair walked up beside me and offered to accompany me past the herd, even though she was going in the other direction. She was on her own with a stocky Jack Russell at her feet.

People are kind, I thought.

As we walked she asked me where I was from.

"North Wales," I said, brightly, smiling at her.

"Ah! My friend is the person who devised a walk up there, based on an ancient pilgrim route. Perhaps you've heard of it – it's called the North Wales Pilgrim's Way."

Yes, I know it well.

It's where my spirit lives.

THE SONG OF GOD

"Arjuna, I am the taste of pure water and the radiance of the sun and moon. I am the sacred word and the sound heard in air, and the courage of human beings. I am the sweet fragrance in the earth and the radiance of fire; I am the life in every creature and the striving of the spiritual aspirant."

Bhagavad Gita, 7.8

MAHAMRITYUNJAYA MANTRA
A MANTRA FOR CONQUERING DEATH:

Om Tryambakam Yajamahe
Sugandhim Pushtivardhanam
Urvarukamiva Bandhanan
Mrityor Mukshiya Maamritat

Rig Veda, c. 1500 BCE

Translation from Sanskrit:

We worship the Lord with the third eye who is fragrant
and who nourishes and nurtures all beings. As a ripened
cucumber is freed from its stem, may the Lord free us from
death, but not immortality.

REVIEW REQUEST

If you enjoyed this book then please consider leaving a review on Amazon, which is the main marketplace for it. It will help its message reach other people who may need to hear it. Perhaps your book club would enjoy reading and discussing its themes of menopause, age-gap relationships, friendships, solo travel, homecoming and belonging, imposter syndrome and reinvention in midlife.

ACKNOWLEDGMENTS

I would like to thank everyone who went out of their way to support me and my first book, especially: Rosie Nixon, Bibi Lynch, Meg Massey, Shubham Komarpant, Caroline Ashford, Simrose Resort, Nick Coveney, Marzena Mizgalska, Clare Baggaley, Mar Dixon, MG Harris, Emily J Johnson, Justin Morgan, Rise Guide (Zoe and Mike), Karen Lloyd, Sarah Searle Anker, Carron Brown, Peter, Gavin and Lynne at Sea Lane Café, Sam Missingham, Gillian Felton, Helen and Steve Peacock, Clair Sharpe, Susan Corcoran, Coreen Ellis, Lucinda Hawksley, Carol Drinkwater, the Bombay Doodler, Sarah Gorrell, John McArdle, Paige Weber, Mandala Café, Sampoorna Yoga School, Kopi Desa, Lily Murphy, Rachel Lawston, Holly, Claire, Jason and Jess Ballard, Aaron Levin, Sunita Ray, Simon Chapple, John Garbutt, Anna Burtt, Emily Benita, Sally Morgan, Emma Drage, Jacquie Bloese, Clara Buckingham and the ladies of the Bayside Book Club in Worthing.

Thank you to *everyone* who took time to write a review, rate or share my book online. It is the most important thing to authors, believe me. Every single one counts.

To my beta readers on this book: Elv Moody, Helen Thomas and Shubham Komarpant – three of the least judgemental people I've ever met who've made me feel good about what I'm doing every step of the way – not just in writing, but in life.

To Guru Gail, who has dealt tirelessly with my emotional outpourings on WhatsApp. You have so much going on in your own life I truly don't know how you find time to help me with mine, but you do. You are a true Karma Yogi and a good friend.

To Miriam Pfeil, who always seems to materialise when I need her the most. Never lose your sparkle.

To David Hilton, Danny and the Cloud 9 Coffee Clinic: mornings wouldn't be the same without you.

To Bram Knuckey and his Chat Room on Worthing seafront – you are an inspiration to us all.

To Marshall, Saluzhina and my Simrose family, for giving me a home and family in India.

To Sudhir Rishi – your effect on my life is unquantifiable but I have tried to do it justice in my books.

Apologies to everyone who encountered Mean Girl or Stroppy Cow over the last decade – I can only hope that this book aids in understanding what happens to emotional control during perimenopause and menopause.

And to all the friends who gave me the space to be silent without judgement for the months that it took to process all of this – I'm immensely grateful.

Lastly, heartfelt thanks to HRT Nurse Karen at Shelley Road Surgery in Worthing and the NHS who dealt with my health scare so quickly and effectively.

Forever in your debt.

FOR SHUBHAM

Some moments that I've had
Some moments of pleasure
I think about us lying
Lying on a beach somewhere
I think about us diving
Diving off a rock into another moment

Just being alive
It can really hurt
And these moments given
Are a gift from time

'*Moments of Pleasure*' *by Kate Bush, The Red Shoes*

ABOUT THE AUTHOR

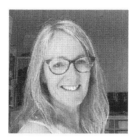

Lisa Edwards is a freelance writer, editor, publisher and yoga teacher. She grew up in North Wales, but lives in Sussex. She splits her time between the UK and India. Scan the code below to access Lisa's newsletter as well as podcasts, interviews and reviews.

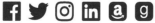

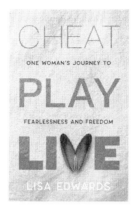

On a beach in California in 2008, Lisa finds a
shell on a rock, its two halves open to the sky.
On the outside it is sea-worn and unremarkable,
but on the inside it gleams like a jewel. It is as
though it is lying there, waiting to be found and
cherished – just like her.

Scan and read more of this inspiring true story…

BECAUSE YOU CAN MINI GUIDEBOOKS
AMAZON EXCLUSIVES

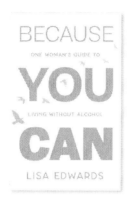

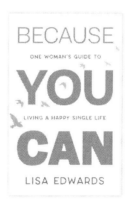

Printed in Great Britain
by Amazon